THE
GIFT
OF
AGAIN

*A Survivor and Caregiver's Guide to
Stroke Recovery and Prevention*

BY YVONNE & TAURA STINSON

Disclaimer

This book shares personal experiences and reflections, along with professional perspectives, including those of medical doctors who appear in these pages. It is not intended to replace the guidance or care of a medical professional who knows your individual health history.

The information here is offered to inform, support, and encourage. Our hope is that these stories provide understanding, connection, and reassurance along the way.

Published by
Dreaming When I Wrote This Publishing
An imprint of Dreaming When I Wrote This Media
Sherman Oaks, California

Printed in the United States of America
First edition

Paperback ISBN: 978-0-692-91481-6
Ebook ISBN: 978-0-692-91672-8

DEDICATION

For Mittie Lee Morton, my mother's mother and my grandmother, and for Adama Wilson, sister-friend-niece. Gone from our sight, but never from our hearts.

First things first. FAST is a life-saving acronym! If you are experiencing any of the symptoms below, please seek immediate medical attention.

FAST – When a stroke is happening

- **F** – Face drooping
- **A** – Arm weakness
- **S** – Speech difficulty
- **T** – Time to call 911

FAST helps you recognize a stroke that is already in motion. It is the tool doctors, nurses, and first responders teach because it can save lives in the moment.

After speaking to several stroke survivors, and in response to my own stroke symptoms, we came up with our on acronym called HEADS UP.

■ HEADS UP – Warning signs in the days or weeks before a stroke ■

- **H** – Headache that is sudden, severe, or different than usual
- **E** – Extreme fatigue that comes on suddenly or lingers without reason
- **A** – Awareness lapses such as confusion, memory loss, or being unable to focus
- **D** – Dizziness or loss of balance
- **S** – Swallowing problems or sudden severe neck pain
- **U** – Unusual mood changes like irritability, depression, or emotional swings
- **P** – Perception problems with vision, such as blurred or double vision

HEADS UP is not meant to replace FAST but to complement it. While FAST helps you act fast when a stroke is happening, HEADS UP gives you a way to notice subtle changes your body may show in the days or weeks before. Recognizing these quieter signals could give you or your loved one the chance to seek care earlier and prevent something more serious

CONTENTS

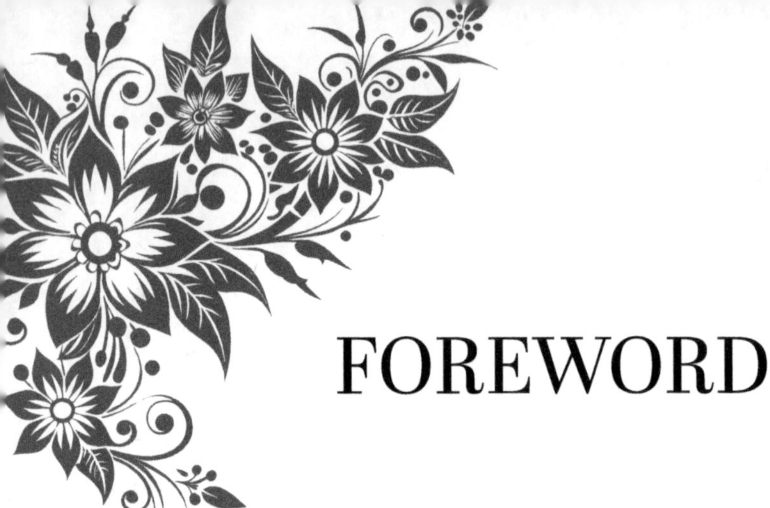

FOREWORD

My Pathway to Neurology and a Tale of Two Strokes

When I really stop and think about it, neurology and stroke medicine have been part of my life for as long as I can remember.

As a little girl, I knew stroke not through textbooks or hospital charts, but through my grandmother. She was loving and gentle, the kind of woman whose presence filled a room. I remember running through her house, past the dining room, and straight into her bedroom, climbing onto her hospital bed and wrapping my arms around her. By the time I was about six years old, she had already suffered a stroke. I cannot remember her walking, but I remember her warmth. I remember her hugs and her soft voice.

I also remember my grandfather and the way he loved her. He cared for her with devotion until her untimely death. She was a wife and the loving mother of ten children, and she was deeply cherished by all of us. Even then, before I understood medicine or illness, I understood love, caregiving, and what it meant for a family to live with the realities of life after stroke.

Fast forward almost thirty years. At that point in my life, I was a third-year nontraditional medical student. I had already fought through multiple failures just to get into medical school, and I had made it past the midpoint. Now I was facing a different question: what kind of doctor did I want to become? When I first entered medical school, I was convinced I wanted to be a surgeon. I liked fixing things. I liked the clarity of it. A surgeon sees a problem and either removes it or repairs it. I am naturally a morning person, and after my surgery rotation, I imagined myself pursuing general surgery followed by a vascular surgery fellowship.

One day, while trying to sort through that decision, I was talking with one of the vascular surgery *attendings*. She was an amazing woman and a phenomenal surgeon. During our conversation, she said something that stayed with me. She told me, "I think you would make an amazing surgeon. But if you find something you love more than this, do that. You have to love this work, because it will ask of you more than you feel is humanly possible."

My next rotation was neurology, and I was scheduled to spend six weeks in the neurological intensive care unit. I saw patients with epilepsy, head trauma, and autoimmune diseases that attacked the muscles and nerves. Still, it was the stroke patients who felt most familiar. Maybe it was because they reminded me of my grandmother, or because I had seen this happen to other people in my community and to those they loved. Whatever the reason, two stroke patients in particular stayed with me.

One patient had an ischemic stroke with relatively limited neurologic deficits. He lost the use of his right arm and had noticeable changes in his speech. In the room next door was a woman who had experienced a hemorrhagic stroke that caused severe neurologic injury, leaving her with very limited movement throughout her body. Both patients had families who were deeply involved in their care, but it was these two individuals who taught me about the power of mindset and will.

The man with the less severe stroke could still walk, move his other arm, and speak, though his speech was slowed and often broken, and he struggled to find words. He was overwhelmed by frustration and convinced that his life was over. He refused to eat and declined to participate in physical therapy. Despite being told that he had a strong chance at a near-complete recovery, he became fixated on what he had lost and said he did not want to live like this.

In contrast, the woman whose stroke was far more devastating was determined to recover, and her family was even more determined. Though she was unable to move, they spoke to her constantly, moved her limbs for her, and included her in every conversation, as if recovery was not a question but an expectation.

By the end of the rotation, the man with the small stroke had grown weaker. He developed pneumonia and was eventually transitioned to hospice care. The woman, by contrast, was talking, eating, moving her arms, and slowly beginning to move her legs. She told me, "I am going to get better," and I believed her.

These two patients taught me a lesson I have carried ever since. While we cannot control our genetics or many of the diseases and conditions that affect our bodies, part of healing lies in what we can control. I saw how mindset changed who showed up to therapy, who accepted help, and who believed recovery was still possible.

This understanding of mindset and the recognition that our brains hold such power ultimately led me to pursue neurology. The brain is the organ that not only controls every other system in the body, but also holds the essence of who we are. Its complexity and capacity for resilience fascinated me so deeply that I could not imagine practicing medicine in any other field.

I often think back to the surgeon who once told me that if I found something I loved more than surgery, I should follow it. Neurology became that path. It is a field where science and humanity are inseparable, and where healing is shaped not only by what happens in the body, but by how patients and families engage with the journey that follows.

When I was asked to contribute to *THE GIFT OF AGAIN*, the reason was immediately clear to me. This book moves seamlessly between memoir and medicine, between lived experience and practical guidance. It is both a deeply personal story and a thoughtful handbook for those navigating stroke, caregiving, and recovery. Seeing Taura and Yvonne Stinson, a mother and daughter, come together to tell this story echoed my own earliest experiences with stroke and caregiving, shaped by my grandmother and the family who surrounded her.

This book speaks plainly about fear, loss, and uncertainty, while also offering clarity, education, and hope to those who need it most.

My name is Kimberly Johnson Hatchett, MD, and I am a double board-certified neurologist. It is an honor to lend my voice to *THE GIFT OF AGAIN*, a book that offers both guidance and presence to those learning how to live, heal, and begin again after stroke.

Dr. Kimberly Johnson Hatchett

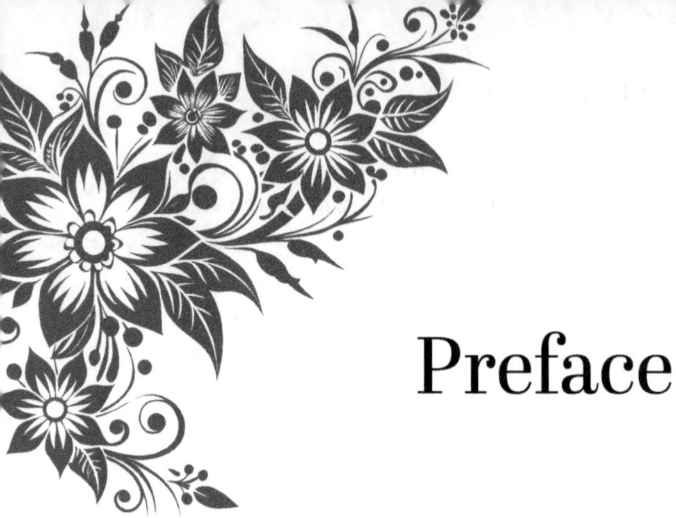

Preface

THE GIFT OF AGAIN

Getting the call that one of your parents has had a stroke is a moment that rearranges you. I had no idea what the next hour would bring, but I turned my wellspring of hope up high and jumped right in. The first word I grasped was *SURVIVED.* My mother survived a stroke. I know that is not always the case, and I was extremely grateful for that. That word became the branch I held onto as I boarded the short flight from Burbank to Oakland. When I arrived, I had to remind my knees to stay still as I approached her hospital bed.

That was in December 2017. December 2025 marks her eight-year stroke **SURVIVORVERSARY.** Eight years of resilience, grace, and new beginnings. In many traditions, the number eight is a symbol of renewal, of what continues without end. For us, it means eight years of waking up again. Eight years of walking, talking, laughing, praying, and loving again. That is the gift of again.

We all know the feeling of wishing for just one more moment with someone we love. To hear their laugh again, to hold their hand again, to see their face just one more time. If you are here, still alive, still breathing, then you are already living that wish. You are the gift of again to someone who loves you.

But *again* is not guaranteed, and that is what makes it sacred. Each moment of recovery, whether it is tying a shoe, hugging a child, or finding your own voice again, is proof of survival and possibility. *The*

Gift of Again is a reminder that life is still unfolding, that healing is still possible, that joy is still waiting.

This book is not just about celebrating my mother's courage. It is about preparing you, the reader, for the realities of stroke: prevention, survival, and life after. It is about what it feels like to walk through the valley as both survivor and caregiver, and what it means to come out on the other side.

Yes, we'll share statistics and sobering truths, because it is important to know the risks:

- African Americans are 50% more likely to have a stroke than white adults.
- Black men are 70% more likely to die from a stroke compared to non-Hispanic white men.
- African American women are twice as likely to have a stroke as white women and 30% more likely to die from one.

And the numbers do not stop there. Hispanic Americans are about 30% more likely to have a stroke compared to non-Hispanic whites. Indigenous people face elevated risks, with some studies showing rates similar to or higher than those in Black communities, and Asian Americans are more likely to experience hemorrhagic strokes. Even among younger adults, stroke rates are rising, leaving no group untouched.

But this is not just about numbers. It is about people. Mothers and fathers. Children, sisters, brothers, and friends. People we cannot afford to lose.

That is why you are holding this book. Our goal is to share our experience along with insights from professionals and survivors, to inform, empower, and prepare you. Inside, you will find recipes, exercises, and practical tools to support prevention, caregiving, and life after stroke. You will also find our hearts, a daughter's perspective, a mother's perspective, and the wisdom we have gathered along the way.

So, grab your highlighter, take notes, and open your heart. May this book help you treasure the most sacred gift of all: the gift of again.

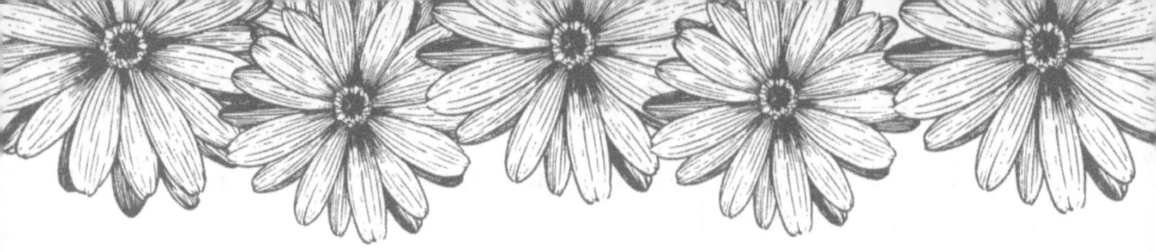

CHAPTER ONE

I'M A SURVIVOR!

Yvonne

I want to first start by Saying how very thankful I am to be an eight-year stroke survivor. Now, my journey includes you. You bought or were given this book for a reason, and we, my daughter Taura and I, are so grateful to be your guides on this journey.

Let's call a spade a spade. What is a stroke? Well, there are a few kinds:

- **Ischemic stroke** – the most common type, caused by a blood clot that blocks a vessel in the brain
- **Hemorrhagic stroke** – caused when a weakened blood vessel bursts and bleeds into the brain
- **Transient Ischemic Attack (TIA)** – often called a "mini-stroke," where symptoms appear for a short time and then go away, but serve as a serious warning signs

In my case, I had a TIA first, which was a *semi-early* warning sign from my body, considering I had a stroke the next day, but some people don't always get that.

I later learned that the stroke that I survived was fueled by family history and driven by undiagnosed high blood pressure. Looking back,

I realize how much my body had been trying to speak to me long before the stroke happened.

I have to say this…even though doctors sometimes label TIA's as "minor strokes," I can tell you from experience that there is no such thing as a minor stroke. Every stroke, no matter the size, is serious and life-changing. A TIA should never be brushed off as something small. It is a HUGE warning sign that deserves all of your attention.

The most powerful weapon we have to fight stroke epidemic is information. Knowing your risks, paying attention to your body, and learning the signs can make all the difference. That is why I share my story with you, so that you or someone you love can take steps before it is too late.

Now for my stroke journey.

It was a normal December day….

But first, a little backstory: at that time, I worked as a teacher's assistant for special needs children, and although I loved those kids dearly, it wasn't easy. That and the rising housing crisis in the Bay Area had me stressed out, in and side to side.

I was a hair stylist my entire adult life, and although we weren't rich, I had no real complaints. However, as my age set in, it became harder to stand on my feet all day. That's how I landed at my daughter's former high school, working as a teacher's assistant. The pay wasn't great, and just a year prior, the home that I was renting was lost to foreclosure, just as the cost of living nearly doubled in the Bay Area. So, I found myself at the mercy of friends, and at that age, I was living in a family friend's home, who, honestly, wasn't the kind of person that should have had a roommate. The stress weighed on me like a coat made of bricks that I put on every day. I had and have a daughter that loves me in LA, and family that loves me in Birmingham, Alabama, and any one of them would have and offered to open their doors to me, but I made my home and planted roots in Oakland, and to this very day, I fight to stay in this place that I have come to know and love, deeply.

Sometime after living with that less-than-desirable roommate, a good friend who had ample space and worked nights mostly offered me a space in his home. It was a godsend. I felt a sense of peace when I moved into his place. I could cook again. I set up my sewing machine and started getting my creative juices flowing, but that coat still weighed on my shoulders from time to time. The weighted stress of uncertainty and not having my own was extremely heavy. Then, work changed drastically. I was assigned to one child at work, and that may sound easier to some, but it was extremely demanding.

After making sure she got onto the bus one day, I slipped on the gravel and injured my knee. I didn't take as much time off as I needed because we were understaffed and they needed me… she needed me! Things would likely have been different if I had prioritized myself, but that was hard because this sweet girl and her mom had become family to me, and I wanted her to be okay, so I needed to be there. That's kind of my thing. I make things better with food and beauty. If you're not feeling your best, come see me for a Red Velvet Cake or a fresh new hairstyle.

Out of my 9 siblings, I was the homebody. The one that stayed at home with my mother while most of my sisters painted the town in vibrant colors. I was in the kitchen with my mom cooking every part of the pig, even the chitterlings. I gave up beef and pork when I was 35, but I will be forever grateful for the time I spent with her, in and out of the kitchen. I cooked alongside her and could feel the weight of her own coat of stress, but she was a southern belle, and southern belles don't tell. Not back then, anyway. There would certainly be no *Real Housewives of Ensely* in the 60's!

She kept house, made amazing meals, and taught her girls and boys how to love ourselves in a world that hated us. We were in the epicenter of hatred, if you ask me. I was born in 1952, so just when I started to understand what life was all about, I was there with my feet planted in the civil rights era. My father gave Dr. Martin Luther King Jr.'s brother the shirt off his back when his house was bombed, only blocks away from where we lived. We witnessed the segregation and "desegregation" of America from our front porch. Funny how some things stay the same.

As I grew up and became interested in boys, I went on a date with a white guy. Segregation was abolished, right? More like, "Yeah, right".

To make a short story even shorter, he took me to a bowling alley in Fairfield, a little town inside of Birmingham, and when we walked in, you could hear jaws dropping, one by one. They didn't say anything, but the silence and hatred was deafening.

We weren't welcome in the bowling alley because of me. Not him. Me.

And that did something to me.

It's important to know the origins of stress, so that you can uproot it. And that was a biggie for me. That and watching my mom suffer emotionally. I was being taught how to manage my own emotions, put on a pretty face, and tuck the pain away.

I didn't date much after that incident, and then I met Taura's father, and although it was such a racist town back then, I thought we'd stay in Birmingham forever. I couldn't imagine a world where I didn't sing with my sisters or get my dresses made by mama, but as they say, all good things come to an end.

It was the 1970's, and I thought things would change, but things only got worse. Taura was hit by a car at 18 months young. It was beyond devastating. After having life-saving major surgery and spending a long period in the hospital, I was pushed to my breaking point. Taura and her Aunt Leila Faye were leaving a follow-up appointment at the hospital when an insanely hateful woman intentionally slammed the door on her tiny fingers and offered a shoulder shrug and half-smile while Faye peeled her fingers from the metal frame. If I needed a sign that it was time to go, that was it for me, so we were off to California!

I thought this magical place of movie stars and a magical mouse would change our worlds, but it did not. What I realized over time is that you can't go anywhere for real change except inside yourself. I've shared a piece of my story to encourage you to go deeper into yours, because knowing the origin of your stress, worry, shame, or whatever it is that keeps you up at night or away from being your best self has to be identified in the line-up. That's the only way to put them away for good, which is not something that I consciously focused on until after my stroke. I encourage you to start that journey now, because stress is a huge precursor to stroke and heart disease.

MY STROKE JOURNEY

Now that you have had a tiny peek into my story, I would like to jump right in and tell you about THAT DAY…

It was a normal December day, but according to various sources, many strokes and heart attacks occur between December and February, but it felt *pretty normal* to me. Outside of my normal stress load, I felt fine at work, but after work, I went to my best friend, Charm's, parents' house to help her father with his comfort. He was dealing with an illness, and she had passed away a few years earlier, due to cancer. Her family has always been my family, ever since I moved to Oakland, and my bond with them grew even stronger after her death. I was fine when I walked into the McElhaney home, but as soon as I sat down, I felt extremely tired. Looking back, it was strange because I wasn't tired at work, while driving, or even as I walked in. But an overwhelming sense of lethargy blanketed me soon after walking in, so I actually slept in the chair for a moment.

NOTE: Pay attention to any changes in your body or your own behavior, and if you can't make sense of it, please seek medical attention.

After waking from a quick nap, I am usually relieved, but I wasn't this time. I was still extremely tired, but I didn't make the safest choice. I drove myself home from Oakland to San Leandro. I can't remember, but I'm sure that drive was with a bobbing head and weighted eyelids, because I was that tired.

When I got home, I made another mistake, but please remember that I am sharing my story so that you can learn from my mistakes.

I got into the bathtub, which no one should do while extremely tired and unsupervised. I always sing in the shower or bathtub, and that night I remember singing "Loving You" by Minnie Riperton. I was still so tired and likely singing to stay awake. And even though I was that lethargic, I had no idea that something was wrong with my body until I felt that sensation. It was like a pop inside my body when I sang the high note of the song. It stopped me in my tracks, but I can't remember getting out of the bathtub. My daughter says I made it to my bedroom because God carried me.

What a comforting thought.

My next recollection is drying off in my bedroom, and while I had intended to walk normally, I found myself walking backward in a circle. I knew it was odd, but I laughed. I didn't know what was happening. I just blamed it on being extremely tired, and I went to sleep when I should have called 911.

Earlier that evening, there was no parking in the area, so when I miraculously got home after DWE (driving while exhausted), I parked at a business across the street. When I woke up from a three or four-hour nap, I looked across the street to check on my car, but I walked backward again, and the laughing stopped. I knew that I needed help. I packed a small bag and walked across the hall to my friend's room, and I thought I stuttered the name of my hospital, but all he heard were sounds that he could not make out. It scared him into immediate action, so he took me straight to the emergency room.

They checked me in, did an MRI, and ran some other tests, but almost immediately, I learned that I had high blood pressure. It was the first time I heard that. If you are reading this and don't know your general baseline, or if you haven't gotten your blood pressure checked in a while, then put this book down and get it checked. Knowing your numbers is so important, and that day, I learned mine. I also learned that I had experienced a TIA.

According to STROKE.ORG, a TIA is a mini (warning stroke). It occurs when a lack of blood and oxygen leads to temporary symptoms such as slurred speech or blurred vision.

There was a time when hospitals would keep you for observation for three days or four days for the smallest things, but nowadays they will put you out before the night is over, like me, just like they did me. I was put on an aspirin regimen and, for the first time in my life, prescribed a bunch of different medications to lower my blood pressure, as well as anti-clotting meds. It was so much to take in, but I faced it head-on. The doctor told me to manage my stress, food habits, and not to drink alcohol or smoke (which I don't anyway), because there is a high probability of having a full stroke within a year of having the TIA. They also highly encouraged me to get a flu shot. It was December, and so many people were getting sick, and I had NEVER had one, but I did that day…then they sent me back home.

I was back at my friend's place just for a little while before it was apparent that something was happening again. I walked backwards and my speech slurred, and then I fell onto a soft patch of fabric, thankfully. So, I went back to the hospital, but this time they admitted me, and I was informed that I had a stroke. This was within twenty-four-hours of having a TIA.

According to STROKE.ORG, a STROKE is a "brain attack" that occurs when the blood that brings oxygen to your brain stops flowing, and brain cells die.

It was time to tell my daughter.

I mentioned before that I learned so much from my mother, and one of those things was not to bother or worry my loved ones with my own problems. At the time, my daughter was going through a once-in-a-lifetime opportunity. Two songs that she had written were circulating in the awards system, and she was bursting with excitement, sharing new magazine articles and exciting updates every day! She and her writing partners had film screenings multiple times a week, and their schedule was tighter than a mosquito's stinger. I didn't want to stop such an exciting time to deal with my issues, but I couldn't pretend to be tired another day when she called. It was December 8th, 2017, when my friend finally called to let her know what was happening, and she was at my bedside the very next morning.

Things sprang into action when she got there. I remember the medical officials giving her a stack of rehab pamphlets in the area, and she toured a few of them within hours of landing. Within a couple of days, I was admitted to one of those centers because I was not a candidate for outpatient recovery. I lost most of the function of my right side and had to learn to walk again. My speech slurred (sometimes it still does) and I just wasn't myself. I'm so blessed to have had her there to choose that facility for me, because all I wanted to do was go back to my own room and get back to life, but life had changed in an instant.

The rehab center is where I took my first steps and had my first physical therapy session, but it was pretty bleak for the first week. Taura and one of her best friends, Adama, were with me most every day, and I attribute that laughter to being as important as the medicine that I was being administered.

If you find yourself in this situation, please don't waste a moment on worry, anger, or fear. It will only ruin your progress. Instead, focus on laughing and sharing space with people who love you and will make you smile. Praying people are important, too, but Debbie and Denny Downers need to be taken off the visit list. Sorry, but not sorry.

It's also important to advocate for yourself and set goals. I asked the medical staff multiple times a day when I could start walking, and I held them to their promise of "soon". Finally, maybe a week into my stay, I got the rhythm back into my stride and started walking again. Taura walked behind me, filming my progress, while the practitioner led me down the hallway. The first time was a bit wiggly, and maybe the third, fourth, fifth, or tenth time too, but like a child wanting to swing at the park, I asked, "Can we try again?" It's important to keep going in your recovery with that kind of tenacity. I have also learned that people who have successful recoveries also have a future date inked, not penciled in. Some dates may be an anniversary, a wedding, or to make a full recovery by your stroke anniversary, but mine was a bit different. While breaking all the rules and lying in the patient bed beside me, my daughter got a call from her publicist, who casually congratulated her on her Golden Globe nomination!

Yes, a GOLDEN GLOBE AWARD, for best original song. We were so excited that I almost skipped therapy to do a praise dance up and down the hallway, but I could only do that in my mind…and "doing that" in your mind is where it all begins.

"Everything is possible for one who believes" – Proverbs 9:23

…and THIS ONE believed! I made a pact with my body, and with God in prayer, that I would be able to go with my daughter to the Golden Globe awards and that I would NOT be in a wheelchair! The very next day, my steps became more confident. I prayed to Jesus for strength and guidance, and I KNOW that He gave it to me. But I am also a firm believer that faith without works is dead, so I worked, and I worked, and I worked, and my body followed the instructions written in my mind and heart.

This is what I did.

REHAB

If you or a loved one has had a stroke, the rehab facility will be your most important step. It focuses on improving mobility, strength, and balance through exercises and activities when possible. These therapies may help you or your loved one regain the ability to walk, stand, and perform daily tasks independently. But it is also important to understand that recovery looks different for everyone. Some people will regain strength, while others may not be able to move at all, and that is not a failure. Therapy is still valuable because it focuses on making life as safe, comfortable, and independent as possible at every stage.

Occupational therapy helps rebuild independence in daily living. For some, this may mean relearning how to dress, bathe, or cook. For others, it may mean learning to use assistive devices safely or adapting the home so that daily tasks can be done with support.

Speech therapy is essential for those who develop aphasia, which is difficulty speaking, slurring their words, or swallowing after a stroke. Slurred speech may occur when one or both sides of the body are affected, whether physically or cognitively, and can make communication very frustrating… Please take it from my mom. Speech therapists help strengthen the muscles needed for speech and swallowing, but they also provide strategies and tools for expressing yourself when words don't come out clearly.

Physical therapy is centered on improving strength, flexibility, and mobility. If movement does not return, physical therapists still play a critical role in helping prevent stiffness, reduce pain, and maintain circulation through guided stretching. Please do not skip this step.

Cognitive therapy is offered when thinking, memory, or problem-solving is affected. Even if mobility is limited, these sessions can help with focus, planning, and communication, giving a sense of control and connection.

Psychological therapy is just as important as the physical side of recovery. Surviving a stroke often brings feelings of frustration, sadness, or even depression. Working with a psychologist, counselor, or therapist can help process these emotions, rebuild confidence, and create coping strategies. This support is not only for the patient but also for family members, who may be adjusting to new responsibilities and changes at home.

Proper nutrition is a cornerstone of recovery, and my mom considers it a part of therapy. Meals at a rehab facility are designed to meet your medical needs first, not necessarily your personal taste, so don't ask anyone to sneak in hot sauce and fried foods. At home, it is wise to mirror that balance with nutrient-rich meals that support brain and body healing, even if they are not what you are used to. Food is medicine now.

A peaceful environment supports emotional healing. For some, this means quiet spaces and rest. For others, it may be uplifting music, prayer, or companionship. Surroundings matter as much as the therapies themselves.

At-home self-therapy looks different for everyone. For some, it may mean walking, stretching, or speech practice. For others, it may mean simple breathing exercises, hand squeezes, listening to music, journaling, YouTube videos, or guided imagery to stay mentally and spiritually engaged. What matters most is consistency and a willingness to keep participating in life in positive ways.

I want you to know that recovery is not a race. It will take time and patience, and sometimes it may feel like you are standing still. I know how frustrating that can be, but with each day you wake up and choose to keep trying, you are healing. Do not measure your progress against anyone else in your life, on social media, at your church, or even within your own family. Celebrate the little victories in a big way. Remember that even on the hardest days, you are still here. If you have even an inkling of determination, the journey ahead will be as smooth as you make it.

Speaking of journey, we read somewhere that it's recommended that a stroke survivor should wait a few weeks before flying, and although there were conflicting reports, we didn't want to take any chances, so my friend gave us a very long and generous ride from San Leandro to Van Nuys, CA. Thank you, Ron!

When we first arrived, it was a bit jarring. Here I am, the mother being cared for by my child. I was grateful, scared, and just a tad angry, if I'm being honest, because although life was stressful in Oakland, it was my life! I had a job, a comfortable little space of my own, and a system that had been in place since I moved there, but I had to play the card that life dealt me and learn to love the game again.

Taura ran a tight ship, and I recognized that the first day. She's an amazing cook who usually makes elaborate meals when I visit, but she followed the doctor's recommendation. She always held up the document, saying, "*Well, the paper says you should…*" The tables had officially turned, and I was the one doing the eye rolling.

There were many things the "paper said," but on this particular day, she was referring to oatmeal. The doctor recommended that I eat Oatmeal every morning to lower my risk of heart disease and stroke and to manage my cholesterol. I also needed a protein source, but not the salty turkey bacon she used cook. Instead, I had to learn to love egg whites, or chicken breasts with Oatmeal, fruit, and veggies. Over time, we jazzed up the Oatmeal and made things tastier, but the beginning was very regimented, even down to what we watched on TV.

Back in my own space, I LOVED watching crime stories and things like that, but Taura would politely turn the station to something sunny and bright. After a while, I understood why, but, whew chile', it was a tug-of-war. She wanted me to be at peace, and I was fighting to regain my independence. She didn't let me take my recovery sitting down either. At that time, the outside of her condo was perfectly circular. So, every morning for the first month or so, we walked in tandem around the circle. First, once around, then after a while, we'd walk twice, three times, and ten times, and eventually, I started walking alone. My car was parked at our family friend Raphael's recording studio for that entire year. Thank you, Ray Ray! And during that time, as advised by my doctor, I did not drive.

I got to know Van Nuys very well because I would eventually walk everywhere. My balance was still a bit off, and my speech was slurred, but I grew stronger and healthier every day as I worked toward two goals. Normalcy and The Oscars!

Yes!

THEEEEEE

OSCARS!!!!!!!

On January 8th, just two days before my birthday, in 2018, I met my first goal to walk, not roll, into the Golden Globe awards! I walked proudly beside my daughter onto the red carpet and into a sea of cameras! I was whisked away to my seat, but I WALKED there. And my daughter did not win the award, but I was so proud of her, Raphael and Mary J. Blige for their nomination for the song, "Mighty River" from the film Mudbound. In the song, my daughter wrote the beautiful words,

"Time tells no lies
It keeps changing and ticking and moving, then

passes by.
But if you're lucky
It will be kind
Like a river
Flowing through time!"
– Taura Stinson

And I was so lucky. So blessed and so proud when just 16 days after flowing like a river at the Golden Globes, I was in my room when Taura burst through the door in tears. She had been nominated for an Oscar! And I knew what I had to do! I had to follow all the steps to recover so I could walk tall into the Oscars and watch her win. And I did, and she did not win the Oscar, but she won as a songwriter from Birmingham, Alabama, who moved to the inner city of Oakland, CA, and defied countless odds to become a celebrated, award-winning songwriter! Yes, award-winning. She won a Critics Choice Award in 2017 for best song in a documentary for the very beautiful song, "Jump", performed by Cynthia Erivo.

I knew there would be more moments like that, and I wanted and WANT to be there, so I did what the paper said and ate salad and grilled chicken when I wanted Enchiladas, and Oatmeal and egg whites when I wanted chicken and waffles, and I walked when I wanted to be in Oakland with the life I built for myself. I prayed when I wanted to give up, I practiced breathing exercises when I felt stressed, and treated every day like the gift that it was, but it was not always a walk in the park. If you or your loved one moves in with someone else, even someone who you love more than anyone in the world, there will be challenges.

I moved into Taura's recording studio room, which was an adjustment for her, and I moved to an entirely new city, which was an adjustment for me. I missed my job and the community that I had built after being in Oakland for most of my adult life. If you or your loved one is going through a transition like this, please go easy on yourself. It's hard to see in the moment sometimes that people just want the best for you. I was so tired of Oatmeal and being reminded to take my medication. Again, it was like a serious role reversal, but sometimes even a necessary change does not feel good. I knew this change was good for me. We spent lots of time at church. Pastor Andrea Humphrey at H.O.P.E.S House was a constant wellspring that we drew from. And I realize that not everyone goes to church, but there's something to having faith. It got me through to the other side, and I highly recommend it.

Physical therapy was a huge part of my recovery, too. In hindsight, it was slow, but so necessary. The PT facility was very close to Taura's condo, and if I remember correctly, I went to occupational therapy for an hour each week and to speech therapy for about the same. There wasn't an option to go more often unless I paid, so YouTube. com became a website I frequented. We researched physical therapy, speech therapy, and followed every rabbit hole to my own personal freedom, and this proved to be a vital part of my recovery.

MY ADVICE TO SURVIVORS

Get moving! That is my advice! Moving physically, emotionally, spiritually and mentally!

After the stroke, every step felt like a victory. Every inch forward was progress. Every muscle that cooperated with my will was a triumph over the debilitating numbness and paralysis that had temporarily taken over my body. It was a reminder of the fragility of the human body and the resilience of the human spirit. The doctors had warned me about the possibility of permanent damage, but I did not accept that. Remember that doctors are people, too, and sometimes they can be pessimistic, but that will not cloud your path forward if you don't let it. Find your focus and keep moving. My focus was on walking. Walking for exercise, walking for adventure, walking for peace, walking for a little slither of freedom and once I started, I vowed not to stop. It may have been slow and unsteady, but it was progress. And I was grateful for it.

My biggest piece of advice to anyone in a similar situation is to walk and talk. As soon as you are able, get up and move, move. And when you think you've walked far enough, walk even farther. The body is a miraculous thing, capable of healing and adapting far beyond what we can imagine. When you are walking, talk. Speak to fear, regret, anger, shame, or whatever is hindering your progress, and tell them all that they are no longer welcome! I huffed and puffed while saying "I can do all things through Christ who strengthens me", as well as other scriptures, because they bring me comfort. What brings you comfort? Talk it through the air that you are so blessed to breathe. After church on Sundays, Taura and I would go to the gym. And we didn't always want to do it, but we kept moving!

If all you have is a hospital room or a rehab center, check with your doctor and get going. Every step you take is a step towards recovery and reclaiming your independence. So don't take it for granted. Embrace it, and keep moving forward. And don't be afraid to ask for help. Surround yourself with supportive loved ones and medical professionals who can guide you along the way. They will be your cheerleaders and your advocates, and they will celebrate each milestone with you, and if they don't…celebrate yourself! Most importantly, never give up hope. Despite the challenges and setbacks, keep believing in your ability to heal and overcome. Because if I can walk again after a stroke, anything is possible!

If you are unable to walk now, fix your mind on getting there. Visualize yourself walking, from how your arms sway, to how your feet feel against the ground, even if all you can do is move your hand… progress starts in the mind and then tells your body what to do. There is so much that you will learn about yourself in this experience, and sometimes it will be extremely challenging for everyone involved. If you are reading this book as a preventive measure, I am so happy for you, and I ask that you take it all in and take it very seriously. We wrote this book in hopes that one day we will not dominate stroke statistics as a people. If you had a TIA and did not immediately have a stroke, as I did, then I hope you are aware that you have the power to turn it around, and some of my advice is still the same: walk it out, talk it through, eat the proper nutrition, protect your environment, and so on. We are not doctors, but our experience, suggestions, recipes, and remedies may help you prevent a stroke, change your lifestyle, and guide you in navigating after-stroke care for yourself or your loved one.

If you are navigating post-stroke care, the journey ahead will be difficult, but it is also filled with opportunities for growth and self-discovery. You will find strength you never knew you had and a resilience that will carry you through the darkest times. The post-stroke journey is unpredictable, but knowledge is power, and by reading this book, you are already arming yourself with the tools to face it head-on. I suggest another good book, one a bit more holy than this one, but that's up to you. However, regardless of religion, speaking life over yourself and your loved ones is something we can all do. Go extra hard on manifesting the best outcome, and it will find you.

Also, please take comfort in the fact that you are not alone; countless others have walked this path and come out stronger on the other side. Their stories, and yours, are a testament to the power of the human spirit…to your spirit! As you turn each page, remember that prevention is key. The choices you make today can shape your future in ways you never thought possible. Small changes, like adopting a healthier lifestyle or managing your stress, can have a HUGE impact on your overall well-being. It is our sincere hope that by sharing our experiences and insights, we can empower you to take control of your health and reduce your risk of stroke. Together, we can rewrite the narrative and give hope to those affected by this life-altering condition. It is a privilege to be one of your guides on this transformative journey. As you navigate the challenges and triumphs that lie ahead, remember that you are stronger than you know. Embrace each lesson, cherish every victory, and never lose hope. Recovery is a marathon, not a sprint, and with each step, you are rewriting your story and inspiring others to do the same.

After a year with Taura, I made my way back to Oakland. The housing crisis and gentrification still weigh heavily on the people who built this beautiful city and continue to love it, but I am grateful to be here. I am deeply thankful for friends who opened their doors and made space for me. Taura and I picked up my car made the drive back to Oakland. My dear friend Dennis became my roommate, and it felt good to have my own independence again, especially driving. After a visit to the DMV to renew my license, as required by my doctor, I had the freedom to drive through the neighborhoods and places that remind me why this city is home to me.

If you have to move away, and then have the privilege to come back home when you have recovered, do not forget to switch your health insurance back to the proper region.

Before I hand it over to Taura, I want to encourage you again to know your numbers. Had I gotten a physical that year, my high blood pressure, rising LDL or other alarms would have moved the doctors or ME into action. The difference between you and me is that you have the information now, and if you are the kind of person who needs a sign, consider this the one.

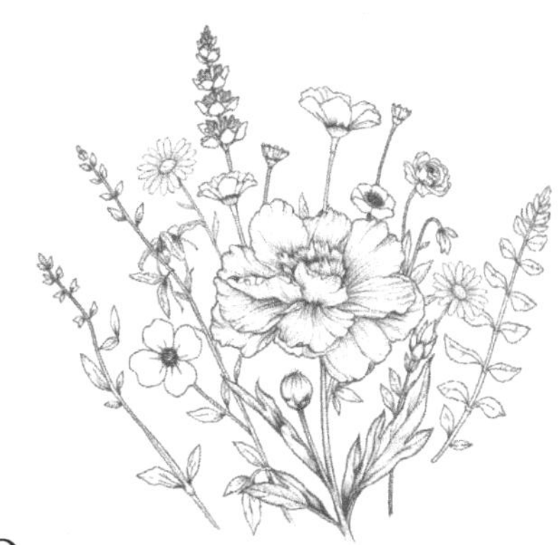

CHAPTER TWO

I AM MY MOTHER'S KEEPER

Taura

My mom and I talk every day, and nothing changed about that on the day that she had a TIA or stroke. She somehow was able to mask her slurred speech as extreme exhaustion, and I fell for it, but I could sense that something was off.

The moment that I was told that my mother had a stroke, my world stopped spinning. I was at a car convention in downtown LA, so fighting through the traffic to get home and throw anything I could find into a bag and immediately hop on the plane was my goal, but I couldn't get a flight out until the next morning. It was the restless night of all restless nights, but I was in San Leandro at her side by 10 am.

And I was a nervous wreck.

My Grandmother, as my mom mentioned, my mother's mother, died of a stroke in her mid 50's. From what I gathered from family conversations, my grandmother held her emotions in, too. Some may have sensed that she was stressed, but she didn't talk about it. I thought about that a lot on the plane from LA to Oakland. There is an old saying that a library burns down every time an elder transitions, and I needed my library....so many books unread and stories yet to discover. I had already left one book unread, and I couldn't bear the thought of closing the greatest and longest chapter in my life.

I was a mess, thinking the worst and ill-prepared, but just before landing, my inner strength kicked in, and I claimed the victory. Manifesting is my superpower, it's actually all of our superpower. The bible says:

Proverbs 23:7 says,
"As a Man thinketh in his heart, then so is he".

And by "he", I know "He" meant "She" too. I serve an inclusive God who loves everyone! So, I stand on that scripture and have done so ever since rising from the smoldering ashes of an extremely challenging time in my life.

I have always believed that words shape our lives. A friend spoke over me with simple, powerful instructions: *THINK. SAY. BE.* I carried those words for a while, but they were not mine. I began looking for meanings that spoke to how thoughts can take root and grow, and that search led me to words rooted in manifestation. Then I came across the words of Buddha: *YOU BECOME WHAT YOU BELIEVE.* Those words clung to me like skin. Among them, I found my own mantra: *BELIEVE BECOME.* I claimed it, lived it, and shared it everywhere from hashtags to tattoos, from emails to social media posts.

But this time was different. I faced a moment where I had to put those words to a monumental task. I could not walk into that hospital room while falling apart. I had to walk in with enough strength for both of us. So, I carried *BELIEVE BECOME* with me, and that is exactly what I did…I believed until she became well.

Okay, now for a little context. My mother is fondly called the Diana Ross of my family. Her hair is always done, her lips bright red, her heels high, and her outfit matching her earrings. So, when I walked into the hospital and saw her in a bonnet, with a natural lip, in front of people, I knew it was serious.

She has this thing where she downplays anything difficult because she does not want to worry me, but in that moment, we were past the point of pretending everything was okay. Well, she was, because I had to hold back the tears that were rising from within and smile at her and tell her that everything was going to be okay, when I had no clue if that were true. *Believe-Become, God whispered.*

Her speech was slurred, and one side of her face was weighted just a little less than the other, but she was still as beautiful as ever. Her skin…brown and flawless, even in her mid–60s, but what worried me deeply was what I could not see. Was her heart okay? Her sister had a heart transplant and would eventually die from it. Is she at risk for that…for another stroke? What about the blood tests, the MRI, the whatwhatawhota.…

I had to hush those intrusive thoughts because I had no room for fear or doubt. Faith needs room to multiply, but if I'm being honest, I was so afraid. I felt like a tree that was shaking so much that my belief leaf had shaken to the ground. My good friend Candace, who lost her beautiful mom a few years earlier, and was a huge help with my mom and me while in LA, reminded me of a line that I had written in a song called "Electric Footprint". The first verse says:

"It's gonna get better. This ain't forever. It's only temporary, it's scary but, if you keep living. Less taking, more giving. It really get's better…swear it's better. In the meantime do what you've gotta do to make it through the storm. You're either going in or coming out…dress warm".

I found myself in the eye of the storm with my mother, holding on to every ounce of strength I had until things could get better. I slipped into the bathroom, looked myself in the eyes, and quietly put on my armor. Just moments before, all I could manage to say was, "Everything's gonna' be okay." But when I returned, I carried questions and suggestions, even as the doctors spoke of her visit days before and mentioned the TIA that I knew nothing about. I adjusted my armor once more and tried to accept that she had kept it from me to protect me.

I did not know what a TIA was, and with the Wi-Fi barely working, it was hard to search for answers. I held back from asking her the questions that weighed heavily on my mind because I did not want to cause her any worry. Instead, I leaned into the still-soft voice inside me that reminded me to stay calm and be her peace.

If your loved one is having a stroke… EMBODY PEACE. If you have had a stroke, please do your best to be at peace. That is a common theme of this book, peace, because the opposite, chaos, turmoil, despair, and the worst of all, FEAR… leads to sickness in our bodies.

I have always been an anxious person, quick to overthink even the smallest things. I was a worry warrior for much of my life, but I am learning to break free from that pattern. As long as I am on this planet, it isn't too late.

I refuse to let worry consume me or dictate how I spend my time on this beautiful earth. Little by little, I am learning to let go, to breathe as my mother taught me, and to trust that everything will unfold as it should. It is not an easy journey, but it's mine! And I am fully committed to making it as scenic as possible for my own well-being. My mother is committed as well, for the very same reason, for her well-being. For OUR well-being.

Now, how about you? Are you committed to not giving any power to the things you cannot change? I sure hope so, because that is where freedom resides!

It was important for me to share that now, because if you or your loved one has had a stroke, or is at risk of having one, chances are you are worried. You may have bought or been given this book because you do not know what to expect. We are here to remind you that, no matter how it looks in this moment, hold on to hope and expect the best.

So right now, before I continue on with my experience with my mom's stroke, I am going to breathe, and I'd like for you to do it with me. My mother taught me this breathing exercise, and it was very helpful to her as she built the tools to worry less.

BREATHE

Please check with your doctor to make sure this is okay, as you may feel lightheaded. For that reason, I do this breathing exercise with my back against the chair or wall and my feet firmly planted on the ground.

Fix your posture and release tension from your shoulders. Now simply breathe in as if you are filling a balloon. Your tummy should expand. Then slowly release it, as if you are pushing your God-given air through a straw. When you are depleted of air, fill up again and repeat the process at least three times.

This exercise does wonders for headaches, recentering and stress management.

The Language of Manifestation

The words we speak carry weight. They can tear down or build up, curse or bless, wound or heal. Science has finally caught up with what faith has always known: words matter. Placebo studies show that the simple belief in healing can trigger real changes in the body.

As you study manifestation like a new language, it is important to set the right environment. Learning a new tongue is not only about practice; it is also about immersion. Surround yourself with words, teachings, and voices that lift you higher. Read books that inspire you, listen to messages that strengthen your faith, and lean into communities that speak life.

For me, certain voices have stood out. Dr. Joe Dispenza's *YOU ARE THE PLACEBO* is a powerful reminder that belief can shift the body and the brain. Dr. Andrew Newberg's research shows that prayer and spiritual practices create real changes in the brain that support healing. Norman Vincent Peale's *THE POWER OF POSITIVE THINKING* is a classic that still speaks truth today about how faith-filled words can open doors. Bruce Wilkinson's *THE PRAYER OF JABEZ* is both a book and a prayer that has been like a blanket to me, one I offer to you for warmth. Sarah Jakes Roberts, in *WOMAN*

EVOLVE, reminds us that no matter what has happened in our past, we can write a new story by choosing words that pull us forward. And Eckhart Tolle's *THE POWER OF NOW* points us back to presence, showing the strength of choosing words rooted in this very moment rather than in fear.

But above all, I return to the Bible. It is the greatest language guide we will ever have. The Scriptures remind us again and again of the power of words. *"LIFE AND DEATH ARE IN THE POWER OF THE TONGUE"* (Proverbs 18:21). *"FAITH COMES BY HEARING, AND HEARING BY THE WORD OF GOD"* (Romans 10:17). *"WHATEVER YOU ASK FOR IN PRAYER, BELIEVE THAT YOU HAVE RECEIVED IT, AND IT WILL BE YOURS"* (Mark 11:24). These verses prove that God has already given us the blueprint.

I know the Bible can be a jarring subject for some, especially when people or systems meant to protect humanity have sometimes done the opposite. But for me, God's Word has never been hard to defend. It is rooted in goodness. Over time, some of its sentiments and messages have been twisted, but the truth remains clear: it is up to us to learn the language of love so we can speak it more fluently. After all, *GOD SO LOVED THE WORLD*…not just certain groups or demographics, but everyone.

As you practice this new language, remember that it is not only about positive thinking. It is about speaking life, speaking faith, and speaking God's promises over yourself and your loved ones. The more you do it, the more natural it becomes, until it flows from you as effortlessly as breath. And when positive speaking takes root, it becomes positive doing, shaping how you show up in the world.

Okay, let me step out of the deep end for a moment and dance a little with nostalgia. When I was younger, my mother guided me to be a dreamer, a creative, and an entrepreneur. She was a hairstylist, as she mentioned, but she also owned a children's party and singing telegram business called *JOYFUL CELEBRATIONS*. My best friend Kyra and my childhood best friend Nioshi know all about wearing those hot costumes in the summer and painting faces for the kids.

She had the kind of faith that moved mountains, and she could dream up things as if she were ordering them straight from a catalog. She hand-made elaborate, spot-on characters like Big Bird, Cookie Monster, Mickey, and Minnie. For her singing telegrams, she created costumes that were bigger than life! A giant heart, a bouquet of roses, even a three-layer cake.

How could I not grow up to be creative and a big dreamer? She had me steeping in possibility.

I also remember hearing her prayers, spoken with such conviction, believing God for things that would eventually come to pass. That faith shaped me, and it still reminds me of the power of the words we speak inside and the ones that make it past our lips.

But even if your speech is compromised or you cannot bend your knees or clasp your hands to pray, know this: what you hold in your heart and shape in your mind, you can one day hold in your hand.

Because speaking life is like learning a new language, here are some language swaps to get started. Try saying this instead of that:

Instead of saying...	Try saying...
I can't do this	I am learning how
I'm weak	I'm getting stronger every day
This is the end	This is a new beginning
I don't know if I'll ever recover	Each day I am making progress
I'm scared	I am covered, and I am not alone
I feel stuck	I am still moving forward, one step at a time
I'm a burden	I am loved, and my life has meaning
I'll never be the same	I am discovering a new version of myself
I'm too tired	I will rest now so I can rise with new strength
This is too hard	This is stretching me, but I am getting through
I am sick	I am healing/I am healed.

Now, I am not going to sit here and present myself as someone better than you. My language has not always been this clear. In fact, I was a serial pessimist who had pockets of realization that I could have what I say, but my environment did not support optimism. What I am about to share is no longer part of my narrative, but it's part of my story, which makes me a different kind of survivor.

I was in two very abusive relationships. The first set the stage for the next because instead of healing in between, I ran into the same arms of the same, familiar monster. In both of those environments, I was unable to hear or see the infinite possibilities ahead of me. Instead, I became the embodiment of the awful things said to me on a daily basis.

My mom is also an amazing poet. After learning that I suffered at the hands of man, just as she had in her youth, she wrote a poem, simply called ABUSE, that deeply resonated with me, especially the stanza below.

> **"You've got to believe that you deserve so much**
> **more Before they demean you to your very core**
> **The Word says, "As a man thinks in his**
> **heart so is he."**
> **Don't allow your ABUSER to**
> **take away your Liberty**
> **Recognize that your power comes from within**
> **You don't have to conform to the ways of a man**
> **Transformation must take place from the inside out**
> **Make positive affirmations and**
> **speak them out loud."**
> **Yvonne Stinson**

The reason I shared this with you is that your environment matters. The things we allow people to say and do to us leave a lasting imprint on our health. You may not be experiencing something as severe as physical abuse, but emotional and mental abuse can be equally damaging.

Stress is not just a feeling; it is a weight the body carries. When stress is constant, blood pressure rises, blood vessels strain, and the brain suffers. Over time, that strain can lead directly to stroke. The mind and body are deeply connected, and what we hold inside shows up in our health.

Prevention begins with protecting your peace. It means setting boundaries, surrounding yourself with people who uplift you, and refusing to carry others' toxic weight. It also means learning healthy ways to release stress, through prayer, journaling, movement, music, or simply taking time to breathe.

When we protect our environment, we protect our health. Choosing joy and peace is not just good for the spirit; it is medicine for the brain and the heart.

Ashé.

CHAPTER THREE

THE CAREGIVER'S HANDBOOK

Taura

My role in this story is caregiver, and a great deal of my time was spent researching. The good news for you is that you don't have to. You can simply take a highlighter and take what you need . I've done my best to gather everything you'll need to be the most prepared caregiver or   caretaker possible.

The first thing I suggest is folding back the page with the breathing instructions so it's always easy to find. You will need it. Breathing, filling your own cup, and doing simple things like eating real food, staying hydrated, and making time for longer showers will make a difference.

Rule number one: take care of yourself. You've heard the adage, "secure your mask first." As a caretaker, that idea is tested daily. You love your mom, dad, husband, wife, child, or whoever you're caring for, but in this season, they are also your patient. Caregiving can drain every ounce of your energy, or it can help you find a healthier rhythm for yourself.

I chose the latter. I ended up losing weight and improving my numbers while caring for my mom. I ate oatmeal and salads and took my vitamins when I gave her hers. When she returned to Oakland, my old habits crept back in. That's why I encourage you to use this time to level up. Caring for someone else can be the spark to care for yourself, too.

The checklist below will keep you organized so you can stay focused on both your loved one and yourself.

Caregiver Checklist for Hospital and Beyond

Paperwork & Insurance

- ☐ Apply for FMLA (Family and Medical Leave Act) or other leave options through your employer as soon as possible.
- ☐ Make sure you are listed as the official point of contact with the care team and the insurance company.
- ☐ Keep insurance cards, ID, and other essential documents with you at all times.
- ☐ Ask about HIPAA forms so doctors can legally share information with you.
- ☐ Begin conversations about bills and financial responsibilities early, even if difficult.
- ☐ Ask about advance directives or medical power of attorney if your loved one does not already have one.

Hospital Care

- ☐ Learn and write down the name of your loved one's primary doctor and key specialists.
- ☐ Introduce yourself to the nurses and staff on each shift. Building relationships matters.
- ☐ Connect early with the hospital's stroke coordinator or patient advocate.
- ☐ Make sure nutritionists, therapists, and other providers know to contact you directly.
- ☐ Keep a current list of medications (names, dosages, times) posted in the room.

☐ Set alarms on your phone for medication times rather than relying on memory.

☐ Cross-check all medications with the doctor to prevent mistakes or overlaps.

☐ Track new symptoms and report them immediately, no matter how small they seem.

☐ Be present during doctor rounds if possible, or request thorough updates when you cannot be there.

☐ Ask for referrals to physical, occupational, and speech therapy before discharge.

☐ Keep emergency contacts written down in case your phone dies.

☐ Watch for infection signs (fever, swelling, redness) and alert staff quickly.

Preparing for Home

☐ If your patient can communicate, ask them where to find important items at home such as medications, clothing, personal documents, or banking information.

☐ Order mobility aids, bathing equipment, and other supportive devices before discharge.

☐ Schedule outpatient appointments and in-home care early to avoid delays.

☐ Create a meal plan with the doctor and nutritionist. Food and recovery are linked.

☐ Plan transportation for follow-ups, especially if the patient cannot drive.

☐ Make the home safe: remove trip hazards, add grab bars and improve lighting.

☐ Pack familiar comfort items like toiletries, lotions, brushes, pajamas, and electronics.

Transfer of Care

If your primary caregiver lives in another city or state, you may need what's called a transition of care. This occurs when recovery takes place outside your insurance coverage area and requires paperwork and advanced planning.

When my mom moved from Northern to Southern California, her health insurance coverage had to be transferred. It took about ten days for the transfer to be approved. That's why you should start these conversations early, at the hospital, rehab center, or even with the doctor when you first meet.

Steps to take:

- ☐ Contact your insurance provider and ask about their process for "transition of care" or "change of service area."
- ☐ Gather complete medical records: discharge notes, test results, therapy evaluations, and medication lists. Request both digital and hard copies.
- ☐ Provide your caregiver information (name, address, phone number, and role) to the care team.
- ☐ Confirm new providers and services in the new location with insurance approval in advance.
- ☐ Ask about timelines. Processing can take a week or longer, so build in buffer time.
- ☐ Double-check prescriptions and supplies to last through the transition.

If Your Loved One Cannot Communicate

If your loved one cannot speak or advocate for themselves, you, as the caregiver, will need to keep their care on track.

- ☐ Establish your authority to act with medical power of attorney documents, or work with a hospital case manager if you don't have them.
- ☐ Partner with the hospital case manager or social worker for insurance guidance and paperwork.
- ☐ Gather all medical records and request both printed and digital copies.

☐ Contact the insurance provider immediately and confirm next steps.

☐ Arrange for equipment like wheelchairs, hospital beds, or feeding tubes to move with the patient.

Packing Essentials for Caregivers (that means you)

☐ Underwear and socks

☐ Change of clothes for 5–7 days

☐ Toiletries, toothbrush, hair products, and any personal care items

☐ Blanket or throw

☐ Cash or credit cards

☐ iPad, phone, and chargers

☐ Medicines you take daily, plus a few extras in case of delay

☐ Medical mask or face coverings

☐ A reminder of your own peace, whether that's a journal, book, or playlist

☐ Something to keep you busy: crossword puzzle, board game, or a work project you can do in quiet moments

Home Setup and Equipment

☐ Hospital-style bed or adjustable bed to improve comfort and ease transfers

☐ Bedpan or bedside commode for patients with limited mobility

☐ Grab bars near the toilet, shower, and bed

☐ Non-slip mats in bathrooms and near the bed

☐ A sturdy shower chair and hand-held shower head

☐ Reacher/grabber tools to help pick up items without bending

☐ Walker, cane, or wheelchair, depending on the doctor's recommendation

☐ Proper footwear (non-slip socks, slippers, or shoes)

Safety and Location

☐ Consider using an AirTag or a similar location device on keys, a bag, or even sewn discreetly into clothing

☐ Make sure the patient's phone has a location-sharing app activated with a trusted caregiver

☐ Keep night lights in hallways, bathrooms, and bedrooms

☐ Place commonly used items (remote control, glasses, phone, medications) within easy reach of the bed

☐ Use door alarms or simple chimes if there is concern about wandering at night

Communication Tools

☐ Whiteboard or notepad with markers/pens for quick notes and reminders

☐ Large-print clock and calendar visible from the bed

☐ Voice-to-text apps on phone or tablet

☐ Picture cards or flashcards with common needs (water, bathroom, food, help)

Emotional and Spiritual Support

☐ Daily routines that include conversation, laughter, or music

☐ Access to faith-based support, prayer lines, or meditation apps if meaningful to the patient

☐ Journaling materials for patients who can write (or dictation apps for those who cannot)

☐ Schedule breaks for caregivers, be it family members or outsourced cargiver's

Personal Preferences

Ask your patient gentle, practical questions to support comfort and dignity:

- Are there foods you dislike or refuse to eat?
- What favorite foods or drinks can be included that also meet doctor's orders?
- Do you have enough blankets and pillows?
- Do you need additional comfort items like over-the-counter medication, supplements, or adult briefs?
- What time of day do you prefer for therapy or walks?
- Can I wash your clothes with my detergent, or do you have a preference?
- Do you have any allergies I should know about?

Financial Discussions

Money can be awkward to talk about, but ignoring it only adds stress.

- Patient's should share bills with their caretaker to avoid missing deadlines.
- Caretakers who cannot absorb additional expenses should be honest. It's okay to say, "Having you here is a joy, but I am on a fixed income and will need to know what you can contribute."
- Contributions could be toward household bills, groceries, or other shared expenses.

Important Documents and Access

Know where essential papers are kept. Ask about bank accounts, property documents, and passwords. My mom added me to her account as recommended by her doctor. We never discussed a power of attorney, but when a friend of mine passed away, her parents couldn't access important accounts or property information.

One option to consider is naming a **POD (Payable on Death)** beneficiary. A POD allows the account to transfer directly to the named person after death without probate. The rules vary by state, so confirm the details with your bank and state laws.

Pencil It In: Linking Calendars

Keeping a shared schedule will make life smoother. I live by my iCal, but my mom preferred a dry-erase board in her room. Both worked. Whether it's apps, sticky notes on the fridge, or text reminders, choose a system that works for both of you. Doctor visits, therapy, medications, and everything else belong on a calendar. The right system prevents last-minute chaos and eases stress for both patient and caregiver.

Resources Available to Caregivers

Due to restrictions with some platforms, I will only share the names of these organizations…please look up the websites.

Stroke Family Warm Line

FMLA (Family and Medical Leave Act)

National Alliance for Caregiving

Family Caregiver Alliance

Eldercare Locator

AARP Family Caregiving Resource Center

National Institute on Aging – Caregiving

Caregiver Action Network

The Rosalynn Carter Institute for Caregivers

Well Spouse Association

The Balm In Gilead

National Black Nurses Association

National Alliance for Hispanic Health

National Indian Council on Aging (NICOA)

Asian American Health Initiative

Closing Notes

Keep all important phone numbers in one place that is easy to access. Including doctors, pharmacies, therapists, insurance contacts, family members, and neighbors. Staying organized will save time and energy when things feel overwhelming.

Check with your loved one's health insurance plan to see if meal services are offered. If they are not, look to your community. Many churches, synagogues, and local organizations offer meal trains or food support for families in need. Accepting help is not a weakness; it is wisdom.

Finally, remember this: not every day will be perfect. Some days will be hard. Some days, you may not get along with your patient, no matter how much you love them. That is okay. What matters most is that you keep showing up, because your main goal as a caregiver is to care.

Whether you call yourself a **caregiver** or a **caretaker**, both are true. You are giving care and taking care, sometimes at the very same moment. And that, in itself, is enough.

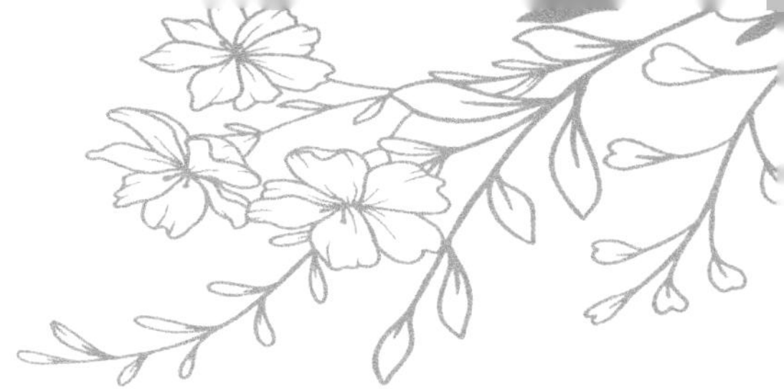

CHAPTER FOUR

FOOD, THE OTHER "F" WORD!

Yvonne

Yes, the other four-letter f-word, that can do some real damage! To minimize the risk of stroke or disease in general, it is essential to avoid foods that can negatively impact cardiovascular health. High-sodium foods, like processed snacks and fast food, can lead to hypertension, which we all know is a major risk factor for stroke. We're from the South, so foods like Macaroni & Cheese, Fried Chicken, and greens cooked so long that the nutrients are depleted are staples, and delicious, might I add.

I jokingly called my Mac & Cheese *Cholesteroni & Cheese*, but in retrospect, that wasn't funny at all. Saturated and trans fats and full-fat dairy products aren't a laughing matter. Neither are fried foods. And don't get me wrong, it may be okay to indulge in moderation every blue moon, especially if you know your numbers, but Soul Food Sunday, followed by leftovers on Monday and Fat or Taco Tuesday, then Hump Day Hamburgers, and so on, could be problematic for your health.

Taura

When we talk about numbers, we're referring to the ones you see on your test results. There are many to consider, but let's focus on cholesterol, since I just mentioned it. LDL stands for LOW DEN-SITY LIPOPROTEINS, and a buildup of these proteins can clog your arteries and increase your risk of heart attacks and stroke. We decided not to recommend specific numbers, because that's between you and your doctor. The important thing is to know your numbers and check them as recommended by your doctor. That's at least once a year for some, but more often for others. We'll talk more about cholesterol later.

NO FINGER POINTING

Von

"It's not your fault. That's something I had to tell myself over and over again. Like, what did I do to have a stroke? But the truth is, if you are anything like me, you just didn't know, and that's a two-part revelation. We didn't know about eating to live, and we didn't know how important family history can be.

My daughter was nearing 10 years old when I started thinking about making lifestyle changes. I'd make wheat germ shakes, likely because that's what was being advertised to me, and we'd go walk around the track at Castlemont High School, but there was a lack of informa-tion out there back then. I was still making beef and pork for dinner, ordering pizza on Friday nights, cooking soul food on Sundays, and Enchiladas or Lasagna during the week was normal behavior. Let's not forget fast food. I was a hairstylist for young people who worked at Taco Bell, McDonalds, and elsewhere, so they showered us with free food. As a result, I started gaining more weight, and so did Taura. I made a drastic change when she was 12 years old. NO MORE BEEF OR PORK.

Taura

That was a big deal for us because it meant no more Beef Stroganoff, Pepperoni Pizza, Cabbage with Salt Pork, Breakfast with Bacon… it was all over, and it made a huge difference in our lives. But honestly, if it had been the magic pill, we wouldn't be writing this book. We have to do so much more and be very intentional about the things we put on our bodies, faces, hair, and in our home environments. So many people live well into their 90s and 100s, mainly due to a lack of exposure to the things that are prominent in today's culture. We didn't grow up wondering how far away the phone needed to be from our bodies at night, or having a plethora of fast, frozen, and canned food options. Those front-facing poisons and carcinogens just weren't around, but now that they are, please, please be mindful.

Von

I know how hard it is to earn a living out here, so I understand *cutting corners*, but the corners are sharper now. Okay, confession. I LOVE discount stores, especially the four-quarter kind, but I have learned to be more selective about what I put on and in my body. Now I go there for greeting cards, balloons, and holiday knick-knacks, not food, lotion, and other mainstays. It's important to know that the same dangers lurk in big-name stores, too. Taura sent me a video of a man making a rotisserie chicken according to the label. Now, I love the roasted chicken from this place, but I had to realize it's not safe for human consumption. The safe option is to keep your eye open for sales, healthier stores, and to wake up early to get yourself a smaller, safer chicken. I emphasized smaller, because I'm learning that bigger does not mean better. Oftentimes, chickens are huge because they have been genetically modified to be that way, pumped with filler, and just other things that shouldn't be in our chicken.

TRANSFORMING YOUR PALATE

Yvonne

The end of this book includes a few recipes that we hope will be extremely helpful to our readers. We have taken some of my Southern recipes and made them healthier. Taura and I were both born in Alabama, but Taura moved to California when she was just 3 years old.

For as long as I can remember, she has been a little chef. I remember that when she was about 10, she made a Diabetic Red Velvet Pie for me. I call it that because she didn't use anything to make it rise and forgot to add sugar. The funny thing is, it wasn't that bad, in theory. So, come with us to the recipe section as we share recipes that may make you say, "hunh??" but taste and see that what the Lord gives us is good! When I moved to Oakland, my former in-laws and I often traded off on Sunday dinners. My house was much smaller than others, but no one missed my dinners. They packed in there and gladly sat wherever they could. The same with Taura. Every time I visit her in LA, she has people gathered around her table like they paid top dollar for it. Her Mexican meals are iconic! She attributes that to being immersed in Mexican culture as a child. Oakland was, and is, a melting pot of many different cultures, and all I can say is Gracias, Bonita.

Taura

Yes, Mexican food is a problem for me. I could, and well, can eat it more than I should. Meanwhile, salads have become a lifesaver for my mom. When she came to live with me after her stroke, a restaurant called La Fogata in Van Nuys, CA, became our second home! My mom faithfully ordered the Grilled Chicken Salad, which is packed with veggies and homemade dressing.

Homemade is so important because processed foods are about the bottom line for companies, not at all about the consumer or our health. The ingredients enhance shelf life and are mostly higher in fat, sodium, and sugar. So be careful the next time you sit down and add processed dressing to your fresh salad. Besides, the taste has NOTHING on homemade dressing! And I get it, it's easier to just buy dressing or tortilla chips or flavored oatmeal, but once you get into the habit of choosing yourself over convenience, you will start to look and feel better.

My mom joked about *Cholesteroni and Cheese*, and mannn, was it good. But our remix version is packed with the good stuff and is a close second to the Southern Mac & Cheese that she and I were both raised on. Was it easy to make this transition? Not one bit, but consider the alternative. The alternative to evolving your palate is staying the same and getting all the things that come with butter, oil, sugar, complex carbs, snacks, fried foods, and all the other delicious things. I laugh when I write this because *good food* usually isn't good for you, and that's subjective, so please don't come for me! I'm sure many will disagree, but that has certainly been our experience until we started playing with recipes and processes to create a new and very delicious normal. But sometimes even the modifications need moderation.

For instance, my mom's famous Red Velvet Cake is usually made with cane sugar. Our modified recipe uses monk fruit sugar, an apples-to-apples substitute that won't spike your blood sugar. Still, it isn't recommended for daily consumption… eating cake every day just isn't ideal. A daily recommendation to satisfy a sweet tooth is to eat an actual apple or other fruit, or add a little cacao or peanut butter to your protein shake. If savory snacks are your thing, an amazing snack swap featured in the recipe section is lemon pepper chips. I always eat them with homemade pico de gallo, but my mom prefers them as is. They are delicious, and people often ask my mom for bags of them. This obsession started when I was little. As a treat, we'd go to a restaurant called "Talk of the Town." They had the best burritos and homemade chips. Because of that, whenever we made Mexican food, we'd cut up tortillas, throw them in a bunch of oil, and slather them in lemon pepper. Although this isn't the healthiest recipe, it's still better than the litany of ingredients in processed chips. However, now when we make chips (and when possible) we go to our local Mexican market and purchase house-made tortillas, looking for the lowest ratio of lard or preservatives. We also choose our lemon pepper and all other dried seasonings wisely. Be on the lookout for those preservatives. They are everywhere and in everything and can be dangerous.

Yvonne

It's important for us creatures of habit to be intentional about our food and exercise habits. We both eat oatmeal almost daily, so we're constantly looking for new ways to make it different and interesting. I love oatmeal with evaporated milk, cinnamon, raisins, butter, and sugar. I didn't miss a beat or notice when Taura swapped evaporated milk for low-fat evaporated milk, butter for Benecol butter, and monk fruit sugar for cane sugar. It's not as hard as it seems, but updating your tools will make this process much easier.

Now, for a disclaimer. We have a list of small appliances that will make this transition much easier for you, but we know not everyone has the money to just up and pay for a bunch of things. If this is you, feel free to use what you have, or consider going to a resale store, FB marketplace, or other discount retailers. Getting everything at once can be overwhelming, which is counterproductive to your wellness, so pace yourself.

And when you are ready, here are the tools that we use, and why.

Air Fryer – Be mindful that the issue health officials have with air fryers is high temperatures. Acrylamide has given air fryers a bad name, but this process can also occur in ovens, toaster ovens, etc. The key is not to over-fry.

Quality Blender – Smoothies and frozen bowls are a great way to pack in fruit and veggies. You might even find one that makes soups and purees, too!

Food Scale – Because portion control is not in the eye of the beholder.

Cast Iron Skillet – A little extra iron and a lot more flavor

Food Processor – You might be just fine with chopping the old-school way, but when your daughter comes over, she cries over your onions. (modern technology anyone:)

Taura

Okay, now that you have your equipment in mind, let's talk food. There are so many things we never thought we could live without, but what I am learning is that I'd rather stop on my own than have it recommended by a health professional. We have both made many swaps, some good and some not so good, but you learn quickly what works and what doesn't. See some of our favorite swaps below.

Instead of...	Try this...
Collard greens cooked for hours in pork fat	Braised collards with shallots, garlic, and olive oil
Biscuits made with white flour and butter	Biscuits with almond flour and coconut oil (or whole-grain drop biscuits with olive oil)
Burgers on processed white bread with beef patties	Plant-based patties or turkey burgers on 100% whole-grain bread
Fried chicken from fast food chains	Air-fried chicken with whole-grain breadcrumbs and spices.
Macaroni and cheese with heavy cream and full-fat cheese	Mac and cheese made with whole-grain pasta, reduced-fat cheese, and blended butternut squash for creaminess
White rice with gravy	Brown rice, quinoa, or cauliflower rice with a light mushroom sauce
Pork sausage or bacon at breakfast	Chicken or turkey sausage, or sautéed mushrooms for a savory side
Potato chips and onion dip	Baked sweet potato chips with hummus or Greek yogurt dip
Fried fish sandwiches	Grilled or oven-baked fish with lemon and herbs
Full-sugar sweet tea or soda	Unsweetened iced tea with lemon, or sparkling water with fruit
Whole milk and cream in coffee	Almond milk, oat milk, or skim milk
Ice cream sundaes	Frozen Greek yogurt with berries and a drizzle of dark chocolate
Processed lunch meats (bologna, salami, ham)	Freshly roasted chicken or turkey breast slices
Packaged ramen noodles	Whole-grain noodles in homemade broth with vegetables and low-sodium soy sauce
White bread toast with butter	100% whole-grain toast with avocado or nut butter
Pastries and donuts	Whole-grain muffins with oats, nuts, and fruit

Instead of...	Try this...
Fried French fries	Oven-baked fries with olive oil and herbs, or roasted sweet potatoes
Store-bought salad dressings (high sodium/ sugar)	Homemade vinaigrette with olive oil, lemon, and spices
Pizza with pepperoni and extra cheese	Veggie-topped pizza on whole-wheat crust with light cheese

The Fat Question

Yvonne

When I first had my stroke, my doctor told me to go on a low-fat diet. At the time, that was the rule of thumb: cut the fat, save your heart. I followed it, and I believe it helped me. Over time, I learned that not all fat is the same. Some fats harm you, and some fats help you heal.

The bad fats are the ones we often crave… the ones we were raised on. Butter, cream, sour cream, fried foods, bacon, fatty meats, and packaged snacks. Those fats clog your arteries and raise your cholesterol. They make it harder for blood to flow the way it needs to.

The good fats are different. Olive oil, avocados, nuts, seeds, and fish like salmon or sardines are the kinds of fats that protect your heart and brain. They reduce inflammation, give you energy, and help your blood vessels stay flexible.

Here's a simple way to remember it:

Bad Fats

- Butter, cream, whole milk, ice cream
- Bacon, sausage, fatty cuts of beef or pork
- Fried fast food
- Packaged snacks with trans fats (look for "hydrogenated oil" on the label)

Good Fats

- Olive oil, avocado oil
- Nuts and seeds such as almonds, walnuts, flaxseed, and chia
- Avocados
- Fatty fish such as salmon, tuna, trout, sardines, and mackerel
- A little dark chocolate

For me, it became less about eating "low-fat" and more about choosing the right fat. And I promise you, once you start cooking with good fats, your body feels the difference. Don't be afraid to try new things. Your tuna fish sandwich doesn't need all the mayo. Your baked potato isn't the problem; it's all that butter and sour cream. And when I say "your," I mean me too. I'm not perfect. I'm over here preaching to the choir.

THE SUGAR TRAP

Taura

If fat was the first villain in my mom's story, sugar has been mine. Sugar is sneaky. It hides in almost everything, not just in candy and cakes. It shows up in bread, salad dressing, flavored yogurt, juice, and even "healthy" granola bars.

The truth is, sugar feeds inflammation. It spikes your blood sugar, weakens your blood vessels, and makes it harder for your brain and heart to get what they need. Over time, it leads to insulin resistance, weight gain, and the very conditions that raise your risk of stroke.

The hard part is that sugar feels good in the moment. It gives you a rush, a sense of comfort, and a memory of childhood. But the crash that follows is a reminder that it is not on your side.

Here's what I've learned:

- **Skip sugary drinks.** Soda, sweet tea, and even fruit juices load your body with sugar it does not need. Water, sparkling water, and unsweetened teas provide hydration without the hit.
- **Read the labels.** Sugar hides under names like corn syrup, dextrose, maltose, and cane juice. If it is among the first three ingredients, put it back.
- **Tame your sweet tooth.** Fresh fruit, a square of dark chocolate, or Greek yogurt with berries can satisfy your craving without the damage.
- **Choose whole foods.** An apple will never betray you the way a candy bar will. The fiber, vitamins, and minerals slow your body's processing of the natural sugars.

For me, sugar has been the quietest yet loudest challenge. I am still learning how to say no to it, but I know this: every time I choose something nourishing instead, I am choosing myself. What's so funny is that I had zero problems with sugar growing up. I ordered grits and potatoes instead of pancakes and waffles and stayed away from desserts, but the more time goes on, I find it harder to resist it. I recently learned that candida could be the culprit. This nice hippie woman who works in the vitamin section at Sprouts asked me to stick out my tongue when I complained to her about sugar cravings, and by the white coating on it, she could tell that I needed to do a candida cleanse. After completing it, the coating was gone, and the cravings and bloating were nearly obliterated.

The Salty Truth About Sodium

Yvonne

After my TIA, one of the first meals I had was loaded with sodium. At the time, I didn't realize how much salt could hurt me. I was tired and wanted something quick, so salt was everywhere in the food I reached for. It tasted good, but later my blood pressure spiked. That was a lesson I will never forget.

Sodium is one of the hardest things to avoid because it hides in so many foods. Canned soups, frozen dinners, sauces, chips, bread, and restaurant meals all contain it. Even foods that don't taste salty are often high in it. One of the worst offenders is ramen. Those little seasoning packets can contain more sodium than you should eat in an entire day.

Here is what I learned:

- **Cook at home when you can.** That way, you control the seasoning. Use herbs, garlic, onion, lemon, and vinegar for flavor instead of salt.
- **Read labels carefully.** Look for "low sodium" or "no salt added." A single serving should contain less than 150 mg, and a full meal should not exceed 600 mg if possible.
- **Rinse canned beans and vegetables.** This washes off a good amount of salt.
- **Watch restaurant meals.** Portions are large, and the sodium is even larger. Ask for sauces and dressings on the side.
- **Remember bread.** It may not taste salty, but it is often one of the biggest sources of sodium in the diet.
- **Skip instant noodles or ramen packets.** If you love noodles, try whole-grain or rice noodles in a homemade broth with vegetables and a splash of low-sodium soy sauce.

I still love flavor, but I have learned to season differently. My meals taste fresher, and my blood pressure thanks me for it. The truth is, you don't miss the salt once you learn to replace it with real flavor.

The Food Myths and Legends

It is easy to be tricked at the grocery store. Labels say organic, gluten-free, plant-based, or low-fat, and we put them in the cart thinking they are good for us. But here is the truth. Organic sugar is still sugar. Gluten-free cookies are still cookies. And low-fat often means high sugar.

Even plant-based can be misleading. Some of the most processed foods in the store now carry that label, from frozen nuggets to imitation meats that read like a science project. If you turn the box over and the ingredient list is longer than the recipe your grandma used to make, it probably is not doing your body any favors.

The key is remembering that marketing sells boxes, not health. Real food does not need a label to tell you it is real food.

Here are some legendary snacks and real foods that will love you back.

- Fresh fruit, especially apples, oranges, bananas, and berries
- Raw nuts such as almonds, walnuts, pistachios, or cashews
- Air-popped popcorn with a sprinkle of herbs
- Greek yogurt with cinnamon or berries
- Dark chocolate squares
- Raw vegetables with hummus or guacamole
- Boiled eggs, ready to grab from the fridge

Everyday staples to stock your kitchen

- Oats, brown rice, quinoa, barley, or whole grain pasta
- Canned beans and lentils, rinsed before use
- Frozen vegetables and fruit.
- Sweet potatoes and regular potatoes…both versatile and filling
- Olive oil and avocado oil for cooking
- Herbs and spices such as garlic, turmeric, basil, cinnamon, rosemary, thyme, and black pepper
- Lean proteins including chicken, fish, tofu, tempeh, and eggs
- Leafy greens such as spinach, kale, collards, or romaine that can be tossed into almost any meal
- Low sodium broths to use as a base for soups and grains
- Whole grain bread or tortillas stored in the freezer so they last longer
- Avocados for toast, salads, or guacamole
- Berries and citrus fruit, which keep well and add natural sweetness

- Unsweetened almond milk, oat milk, or skim milk
- Cottage cheese or reduced fat cheese in small portions

Freezer and fridge helpers

- Bags of frozen berries for smoothies or oatmeal
- Frozen fish fillets like salmon or cod that can be baked quickly
- Frozen brown rice or quinoa packets for fast meals
- Chopped frozen spinach or kale to add to soups, eggs, or pasta
- Plain frozen edamame for a high protein snack

When your kitchen is filled with foods that love you back, eating well becomes less about restriction and more about building habits that help you thrive.

THE CASE FOR PLANT BASED

In preparation for my annual physical, I decided to go vegetarian. I will be real with you; it takes discipline. If you are like me and love crunchy fried fish and chicken, making changes can feel like a tall order. Change is not always easy, but consider it a privilege to make the shift before your doctor tells you that you need medication.

For a month, I drank the *HOW LOW CAN YOU GO* shake from the recipe section. I basically put the lion's share of daily recommendations from the book *CHOLESTEROL DOWN* into a shake, along with the protein of my choice. I also had Sola toast with plant sterol butter and swallowed one whole clove of garlic each morning. Side note: if you have not read *CHOLESTEROL DOWN*, please get it. It is filled with life-saving information. It is by Janet Bond Brill.

Six months prior, my bad cholesterol (LDL) was high, as were my triglycerides. The LDL had crept up over the years, first to 117, then into the 130s, and finally to 155. That one scared me. Again, these are my numbers, not yours, so check with your doctor about what is high or normal for you. But for me, it was alarming. I had made significant changes, even losing 60 pounds, but I guess I was not as cute on the inside as I was on the outside. The scale was going down, but my numbers were creeping up.

I remembered reading that while genetics play a role in cholesterol and heart health, we can often influence and even reverse hereditary risk through consistent lifestyle changes. Research from Harvard Health and the Cleveland Clinic has shown that diet, exercise, and stress management can affect how certain genes linked to cholesterol are expressed. In other words, what we eat, how we move, and how we care for our emotional health can change how our body responds. Most people can begin to see improvement within six to eight weeks of consistent dietary changes, though it may take a few months for lab results to fully reflect those changes.

I exercised more and got my protein from plants, legumes, tofu, and other plant-based sources. I was not fully vegan because I still ate fat-free Greek yogurt and the occasional Parmesan cheese, but everything else had major swaps. I even had a mini funeral for sour cream, lol. I would still eat my famous bean and cheese burrito, but now the cheese was plant-based, and the sour cream was fat-free Greek yogurt mixed with taco seasoning and cilantro.

I am now very proud to say that my numbers have improved dramatically. My LDL dropped from 155 to 82, and my triglycerides fell to 57. I do not recall the exact starting number, but I know this: the inside finally matched the outside, and that felt better than any number on a scale ever could.

My life plan is to eat mostly plant-based. Even yogurt is getting a makeover as I try new options to replace dairy. This is where my life plan becomes flexitarian. While I mostly avoid dairy, I eat fish twice a week. I also leave the door cracked open to chicken, but in the same way that I enjoy ice cream, only every blue moon, on my birthday, or during holidays.

I am learning to listen to my body all over again, and I know this is something I can stick to. I have made that agreement with myself. What agreement are you making or planning to make with yourself? If it includes being vegan or vegetarian, make sure you have plenty of protein sources. Below are some solid options. The key is variety. Mixing beans, grains, seeds, and nuts gives your body what it needs to stay strong, satisfied, and balanced. Here are some of my favorites:

- Soybeans
- Tofu
- Tempeh
- Edamame (young soybeans)
- Lentils
- Black beans
- Kidney beans
- Chickpeas
- Lima beans
- Black eyed peas
- Green peas
- Oats
- Quinoa
- Hemp seeds
- Chia seeds
- Pumpkin seeds
- Pistachios
- Almonds

If you are just starting out, try adding one or two of these to each meal. Over time, your plate will begin to look and feel balanced.

It can be a lot to take in if this feels completely new, but you really cannot knock it until you try it. Every time you swap meat for one of these options, you are not only eating differently, you are also giving your heart and brain another layer of protection. Over time, those small shifts add up and begin to feel natural.

THE GOOD, THE BAD, AND THE UGLY ABOUT MEAT SUBSTITUTES

When I first started exploring meat alternatives, I thought I had struck gold. There were so many options that looked and tasted like the real thing, but I quickly learned that not all substitutes are created equal. Some can support your health goals, while others are just highly processed versions of what you are trying to move away from.

The Good

The best meat substitutes are made from whole, plant-based foods. These include lentils, beans, mushrooms, chickpeas, tofu, tempeh, and seitan. They are naturally high in protein, low in saturated fat, and rich in fiber, helping you feel full longer. You can season and cook them creatively, and your body will thank you for keeping things close to the earth.

The Bad

Some packaged meat alternatives are marketed as healthy but are loaded with sodium, oils, and preservatives. Many popular options use ingredients that are difficult to pronounce or unnecessary for something meant to nourish your body. Always read the label. If it has more than ten ingredients or sounds like a science project, again, it may not belong on your regular grocery list.

The Ugly

Then there are ultra-processed products that may look like burgers or nuggets but are loaded with artificial flavors and additives. These can raise your cholesterol and blood pressure just like regular fast food. A good rule of thumb is that imitation meat should not be your main source of protein. Think of it as a convenience food for a busy day, not an everyday meal.

Taura's Favorite Clean Brands

When it comes to store-bought options, a few brands do it better than others. These are the ones I reach for when I want something quick but still mindful of ingredients.

- **Hilary's** – Veggie burgers and breakfast patties made with whole grains and real vegetables, not fillers.
- **Dr. Praeger's** – Simple, recognizable ingredients you can actually see. The California Veggie Burger is a classic for a reason.
- Gardein Ultimate Plant-Based Fillets – A good option when you want something hearty and familiar but still lighter than traditional fried food.
- **Abbot's Butcher** – Clean, soy free, and made from pea protein with a short ingredient list you can read without a science degree.
- **Daring** – Simple, minimally processed chicken-style pieces made mostly from soy protein, great when you want texture without additives.
- **Actual Veggies** – Thick, colorful patties made from real vegetables, grains, and legumes. No artificial meat flavor, just honest food.
- **Field Roast** – Flavorful sausages and roasts made with grains, vegetables, and real herbs. High in protein, satisfying, and one of the few plant-based meats that actually feels like a meal rather than a substitute.

Store Brands

- **Trader Joe's High Protein Veggie Patty** – Balanced flavor and great texture, made with pea protein instead of mystery ingredients.
- **365 by Whole Foods Market** – Their plant-based patties and veggie burgers are made with whole ingredients such as beans, lentils, and grains. A reliable and affordable choice for quick, nourishing meals.
- **Sprouts Brand Plant-Based Burgers and Sausages** – Made mostly from pea protein and vegetables, with fewer additives than

most national brands. Their spicy Italian and mushroom versions are especially good.

Even if brands change or become unavailable, the message does not. The closer your food is to its natural form, the better it will serve you. A simple rule of thumb is to choose foods with ingredients you recognize, words you can pronounce, and colors that come from nature. If it started as a bean, grain, or vegetable, you are on the right track. Whole foods always win.

GLP-1's

Now, a brief word about GLP-1s and my personal journey.

At first, I wasn't going to talk about how helpful these medications have been in my fight against obesity. But they are part of my story, and I am proud to own all of it.

When I first started on a GLP-1, I did lose a significant amount of weight, but quite honestly, it made me very sick. My doctor made adjustments, but it just was not working for me the way it does for some people. I lost about twenty pounds quickly, but I earned every single one of those pounds through serious lifestyle changes and hard work.

My nurse practitioner, Jessica Brewer, talks more about this later in the book, but my advice to you is simple. Research it. Do not just read the headlines. Learn what works best for your body. Even then, whole foods, moderation, and paying attention to your sugar, sodium, and fat intake matter so much.

Are GLP-1s a magic shot for some people? Absolutely. Some bodies respond to them beautifully, inside and out. Mine did not. It took a lot of work and a lot of adjustments with my medical team, just like managing any other disease.

I felt deeply seen when I watched Oprah's special on obesity as a disease because I often feel like I did not earn this body. I know that sounds strange, but it is the truth of how I feel. I tried every diet and often had the worst results. I grew up loving to cook and eating rich, flavorful food, yet I had friends walking beside me in size-five bodies who could eat me under the table.

After lowering my LDL and losing sixty pounds with the help of GLP-1s, I decided to give my body a break. Maybe I had been on them too long. For full transparency, they were also incredibly expensive. As a creative living in a world where greenlights can turn red overnight, I simply could not afford them anymore.

I am writing this now, twelve pounds heavier. I recently lost three pounds after restarting tirzepatide. When I spoke to my general practitioner, his advice was clear. I needed to start again. I was scared to commit to a medication that could be part of my life long-term. He said, "The benefits outweigh the risks."

So yes, food may feel like the other F word, but so is fn' obesity!

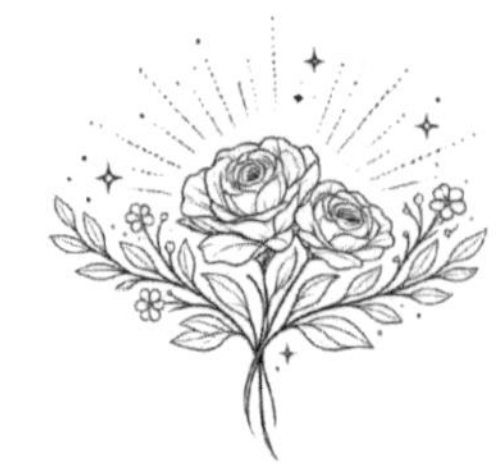

CHAPTER FIVE

SURVIVOR VERSES

Taura

Every stroke survivor carries a verse in a larger song of resilience. No two verses are the same, yet together they create a harmony of survival, hope, and renewal. This chapter is not about statistics alone, though they matter, nor only about medicine, though it saves lives. It is about the personal experiences of stroke survivors who turn their pain into testimony. Each story here is a verse, and when read together, they form a chorus of healing.

We've decided to include the stories of other stroke survivors in the hope that you, the reader will connect with someone whose stroke may not have looked like my mom's. Maybe you will connect more with male storytelling or with the experiences of younger people. Whatever the case, our hope is that you find a voice here that feels familiar enough to remind you that you are not alone.

These pages bring together survivors from diverse backgrounds, each sharing how stroke shaped their journeys, their families, and their healing. No two strokes are the same, and no two survivors respond the same way. Yet when these stories are placed side by side, they create a path of light for others to follow.

Clarence McElhaney: Grief, Grace & Gratitude

Von

First up, we talked to my brother from another mother, Clarence McElhaney. The McElhaney family became my family through my late best friend, Chauming McElhaney. We called her Charm, and she was just that. I had lived in California for some time before Charm and I became friends. We met at church and became inseparable at a time when I needed it most. My ex-husband and I were divorcing, so it was just me and Taura. That became painfully obvious as the invitations we used to get from her dad's family became far and few between. That is when the McElhaney's stepped in. Mrs. Mac opened her doors to us through her daughter, and we became family. We were invited to all of the family gatherings and found a sense of peace amid the chaos of divorce. I was there when Charm became mom to three beautiful children, and I was in her home when she took her last breath. Following her transition, my connection with the McElhaney's deepened. I certainly look at Ms. Mac as a second mom and all of the McElhaney men as brothers. In fact, I was at the McElhaney's, sitting with Mr. Mac while he was sick, as I first started showing signs of a stroke. Years later, we spoke to the brother closest in age to me about his own stroke journey.

On March 10, 2019, Clarence and Lynette's only son, Victor, was killed while away at college. When asked whether he thought that may have played a role in his stroke, Clarence said it was highly plausible. Due to the pandemic and other circumstances, it took five years to prosecute Victor's murderer. For Lynette and Clarence, that period must have felt like living with the screen door cracked open on grief, never able to close it fully. It was hard to watch, and because of my own recovery, I had to pace myself. Taura, however, was there with them at the hospital and throughout the process.

Victor was a gifted young man who could play the skins off any drum. We were blessed to watch him grow from a child into a man finding his own way. His life was vibrant, and his presence continues to inspire.

The weight of grief cannot be overstated. Studies show that the death of a child dramatically increases the risk of cardiovascular events. Research published in the Journal of the American Heart Association found that bereaved parents were nearly twice as likely to suffer a stroke or heart attack in the first year after loss, with the risk peaking in the first thirty days. Other studies confirm that grief is not only emotional but also physical. It disrupts sleep, raises blood pressure, increases clotting, and floods the body with stress hormones that strain the heart and blood vessels.

Clarence shares how this truth lives in him. Losing Victor is more than an emotional wound. It is a heaviness pressing into his body. He describes grief as something that takes up residence inside you, something that can weaken you if you are not careful. The years of waiting for justice only deepen the strain, stretching grief into a long shadow that feels impossible to step out of.

Grief is not only emotional; it is physical, and its toll on the body is both silent and profound. Check in with your body. If you need medical attention, do not delay seeking it.

Clarence's stroke came quietly in the middle of the night. "I just did not feel right," he says. "I could not explain it. Something was off, so I told Lynette, I think I need to go to the doctor." Though he is still able to walk, talk, and even joke with the paramedics, he trusts his instincts. At the hospital, an emergency physician decides to keep him overnight. Testing later confirms that Clarence has suffered a small stroke, one that might have gone undetected had he ignored his body's signals.

At sixty-five, Clarence considers himself fortunate. His right side is slightly weaker, but he remains independent. "I know men my age who had strokes and cannot walk," he says. "Mine was smaller, but it made me pay attention."

About one in three people who have experienced a TIA, or ministroke, will go on to suffer a more serious stroke within a year, often within the first few days.

Even the briefest interruption of blood flow can cause damage, and every stroke is a warning sign that should be taken seriously.

After his stroke is confirmed, Clarence reflects on the health challenges he had already been carrying. Diabetes is one of them, and he often speaks about the frustration of living with a condition that seems to follow him everywhere.

Research shows that people with diabetes are twice as likely to have a stroke as those without diabetes. High blood sugar damages blood vessels over time, increasing the risk of clotting and narrowing the arteries. This makes strokes not only more likely but often more severe.

Clarence believes that connection explains part of his own story. "It is all tied together," he says. "You cannot separate the stress from the grief, the food from the medicine, or the diabetes from the stroke. It is all one body. If you do not take care of it, something will break."

For Clarence, that realization became motivation. He began looking for ways to lower his blood sugar that did not rely solely on prescriptions. His A1C, which had been stuck at eleven, begins to drop. Within months, he sees it fall to nine, progress he had never achieved with traditional medication. For him, that number is not just about what he puts into his own body. It is proof that he continues to lower his risk of another stroke and protect himself against a heart attack as well.

"Even if you eat organic, our food is toxic," he explains. "The water, the soil, everything. We live in a very toxic environment." He speaks passionately about how the food system has changed. "There are countries where people live to a hundred. They drink, they party, they eat rice three times a day. They do not have the problems we have. It is something in the way we live here."

Blue Zones research shows that centenarians around the world live longer, healthier lives by eating mostly plants, beans, and whole foods, staying active daily, and maintaining close social and community ties.

Clarence believes this is proof of what he already senses. "They eat simple food and they move. That is the secret. Here we have all these preservatives and chemicals. The body was not designed for that."

Dr. Valter Longo's research expands this picture. His studies on fasting and longevity show that cycles of fasting and a primarily plant-based diet can reduce inflammation, lower blood sugar, and trigger cellular repair. Longo's work suggests that the body has built-in healing programs that can be switched on when we stop overloading it with processed foods and constant eating. In Blue Zones, where people regularly live past one hundred, many of these patterns are present: small meals, long breaks between them, reliance on whole plants, and a rhythm of life that prioritizes community and movement.

Clarence's Tools for Healing

Clarence's story is both deeply personal and practical. He believes healing is not only about medicine but also about listening to your body, managing stress, and leaning into the natural tools God has already provided.

Holistic Supplements and Alternatives

- Sea moss to help lower blood pressure
- Black seed oil for circulation and overall health
- Apple cider vinegar tablets as a gentler option than drinking it directly
- Cinnamon concentrate to support blood sugar control
- Blood Level Maintenance (BLM) to regulate blood sugar
- Blood Sugar Detox at night to support the pancreas

Clarence speaks about these with the same seriousness most people reserve for prescriptions. He does not see them as magic bullets but as supports that help the body function as it was designed to. "It is about consistency," he says. "Take care of your body every day, not just after you get sick."

Dietary Shifts

- Fresh berries daily, including blueberries, blackberries, and raspberries
- More fish while staying mindful of mercury
- Occasional red meat with a focus on quality and moderation
- Reduced gluten to support digestion and inflammation
- Avoided processed foods and unnecessary sugar

Lifestyle and Exercise

- Chair cardio and light movement to maintain circulation
- Gradual return to walking in nature, wearing supportive shoes if you can.
- Stress management and emotional pacing.
- Daily focus on whole foods, hydration, and consistency
- Rest and proper sleep

Clarence also speaks about how men often dismiss their symptoms until it is too late. "Men think if they can still stand up, still drive, still go to work, then nothing is wrong," he says. "But we cannot keep ignoring what our bodies are telling us. That is why I went to the doctor that night. I was not going to gamble with my life."

Words of Wisdom

Clarence's reflections are not just about his own survival but about how to live better. He urges people to trust their instincts because the body always signals when something is wrong. He wants others to believe that no diagnosis is permanent and that healing is possible if you give the body what it needs. He encourages movement, foods that give life rather than deplete it, and patience with the process. He reminds us that medical advice has its place, but God also provides natural supports that should not be ignored. Clarence teaches that grief and stress can harm as much as a poor diet, and he urges everyone to manage both with care and intention.

He is also clear that his story is not just about him. Lynette, his wife, is his anchor and his powerhouse throughout it all. Together, they carry the weight of unimaginable grief while holding on to faith and to each other. Clarence calls her his strength, and watching them together is proof that resilience is magnified by love.

Closing Note

Clarence's journey is a reminder that recovery looks different for everyone. His strength reflects not only his own choices but also the love of his family and the memory of his son, Victor, whose life continues to inspire resilience and hope. And standing beside him through it all is Lynette, a testament to the kind of partnership that makes survival not only possible but also beautiful.

Emiko Carlin: WHEN THE BEAT DROPS

I was excited when Emiko agreed to be part of this book because we live in the same musical world. There was an immediate sense of recognition between us, the kind that happens when you know the language someone else speaks without having to explain it.

Talking to Emiko was like catching up with a very close friend. We just fell right in, even though we had just met moments earlier.

She is a musician, a composer, and a singer-songwriter, and part of my life's work is to shine a light on women like her. Like us. Women who continue to create, even when their bodies and their spirits have been tested. Women whose stories hold more than one rhythm at a time.

Through Emiko, I get to do that in many ways, including introducing her advocacy, her upcoming documentary, and her role as a musical force to all of you. However, today, the light shines on Emiko as a three-time stroke survivor and heart attack survivor, whose story asks us to pay closer attention and advocate for ourselves.

As Emiko shared her story, it became clear that the warning signs did not arrive in a way that demanded immediate attention. They did not interrupt her life with urgency or spectacle. They arrived quietly, folded into the shape of her days, easy to explain away as stress, exhaustion, or the normal strain of a creative life lived at full speed.

Her first stroke was a TIA, and it happened in her late thirties. At the time, it did not look the way people expect a stroke to look. There was confusion. A sense that her thoughts were slightly out of sync with her body. Words felt harder to reach, focus came and went, and her body felt unfamiliar in subtle but unsettling ways. Nothing dramatic enough to stop her day, but enough to register. She noticed it, and, like many women who function through discomfort, she kept just going. Her first stroke was a transient ischemic attack, or TIA, and it happened at NAMM, a yearly music tech conference in Anaheim where performing is a very big deal. Emiko had a headache that at first did not seem unusual. At NAMM you are performing in front of peers and people you may admire, so some stress and tension feel normal. But the pain became so intense that she ended up in the ER, where it was dismissed as nothing more than a headache. This was January 16th, 2020, and shortly thereafter, Covid brought a nationwide shutdown, making immediate follow-up nearly impossible. It was later confirmed by her physician, with a neurologist in agreement, that she had in fact experienced a TIA. If you have been reading this book, then you already know that a TIA is no small thing. It is a blaring warning that the risk for a future stroke is significantly higher. And she was at higher risk. But she had not made any of the changes that might have helped prevent what came next, likely because no one told her she needed to. Let Emiko's story be a reminder that we are allowed to ask as many questions as we want and self-advocate, because warnings are signs of danger ahead.

In November of 2022, Emiko was sitting at the kitchen table at home during an otherwise ordinary evening, with her then-partner, with the television on, and just eating ice cream. Then what felt like a relaxed night took a sharp turn. Something shifted. Not pain, but a sudden internal knowing that something was wrong. She did not feel like herself. Her body felt unfamiliar again. She told her then-partner that she did not feel well and thought she should go upstairs and lie down, but thankfully, he didn't let her. Within moments, she was having a full-blown stroke, and would have certainly died had she gone upstairs.

In an instant, she was on a gurney in the emergency room. What had once been a warning returned, louder this time, leaving no room for dismissal from medical professionals. At the hospital, things moved quickly, but one figure stood out to Emiko as everything blurred around her. As she was assessed and moved through the emergency room, drifting in and out, a Black man with a beard appeared at her side. He was calm and steady, speaking to her with assurance and care. On the gurney, Emiko kept repeating one phrase. "Somebody help me" without realizing that she wasn't speaking coherently. She had temporary aphasia as a result of the stroke, but someone heard her clearly. His presence brought her comfort in a moment when her body felt completely out of her control. This time, the warning could not be overlooked. Tests were ordered. Specialists were called in. What emerged was not a mystery but missed information. Emiko was eventually diagnosed with premature ventricular contractions, a condition in which the heart beats too many times and too irregularly. Over time, that constant misfiring had frayed a valve in her heart, allowing tiny clots to form and travel upward. Those clots had been the source of her strokes. Surgery followed, along with the placement of a heart monitor designed to track the very rhythm her body had been trying to flag for years. For the first time, there was clarity. Not comfort, but understanding. And with it, the beginning of a real path forward.

Emiko's faith was restored as well when she later learned that no Black man, with or without a beard, had been on staff at the hospital that night. No one could account for his presence. What she remembered so clearly did not appear on any chart or schedule. Maybe angels do wear scrubs after all.

The third event came after the surgery, which made it so unsettling. By then, Emiko had done what she was told. She had the procedure. She was being monitored and had even lost sixty pounds. She believed the worst was behind her. But bodies are complex, and healing is not always linear. In the days leading up to it, she noticed familiar signals returning. A burning sensation she tried to explain away. Fatigue that felt heavier than usual. A pressure in her chest she assumed was stress. She had learned how easy it was to minimize herself, even after everything she had survived.

The heart attack came first. Later that same day, a second TIA followed. She was in Las Vegas when it happened, which she now calls a grim kind of combo. What stands out is not just the severity but her awareness. She remembers the sensation of being underwater, the sweating, the inability to breathe, and the moment she realized something was deeply wrong. Even then, instinct kicked in. She pulled her car over. Yes, this superwoman was driving. She was headed to a meeting she felt she could not miss, and she went anyway. But when she arrived, a friend took one look at her and urged her to seek medical care. She is grateful she listened. What Emiko later learned was that the device implanted during her surgery was designed to monitor a specific heart rhythm issue, not to prevent every possible cardiac or vascular event. The surgery addressed one problem, but it did not erase the impact of prolonged stress, trauma, and a body that had spent years in fight-or-flight.

Recovery this time was different. Not because it was easier, but because Emiko was different. She was informed. She no longer felt obligated to soften her needs or explain her limits. Her patience for nonsense had evaporated. What emerged instead was a mantra that makes her laugh and keeps her alive. "Mother f**ker, back up." It is not about anger. It is about boundaries. It is about protecting her nervous system, her peace, and the body that has already fought harder than most. She no longer negotiates with exhaustion or dismisses warning signs. She listens, and she is not afraid to ask for help when she needs it.

In closing, I want to highlight Emiko's documentary, *Code Stroke*, which is currently in production. The film centers on young stroke survivors and examines what happens when warning signs are missed, care is delayed, or patients are forced to advocate for themselves in systems that are not built to listen. Through the stories of survivors, doctors, and caregivers, *Code Stroke* pulls back the curtain on recovery, resilience, and the invisible aftermath of stroke. It is advocacy born of falling three times and getting back up stronger, again.

Out of everything she has endured, advocacy has become her clearest offering. Telling these stories has become part of her healing, a way to make meaning of what almost took her. Emiko continues to create, compose, and write music that carries all of this with it. Her life now holds more intention, more honesty, and more rest. Her story reminds us that survival is not just about getting through the crisis. It is about learning when to stop, when to speak, and when to say, without apology, motherfu★★er back up.

In music, the drop is not the end. It is the shift that gets the party started. When the beat dropped in Emiko's life, it became the moment she learned to listen and two-step to the rhythm of her own becoming, leaving everything else a step behind.

Tracey Brown: Be healed and Rise!

Taura

When I met Tracey Brown, I didn't just meet a survivor. I met walking sunshine! She is light in motion, proof that faith can find its footing in the darkest places. A stroke and breast cancer survivor, she turned her pain into purpose and her healing into a lifestyle. Every word she speaks carries the weight of someone who has been tested and transformed.

At thirty-seven, Tracey was living her purpose through movement. Known as ***BodyTraceFit*** in Cleveland, she was traveling, teaching, and competing at the top of her game. Fitness wasn't a job for her; it was a ministry. "Tracey was the one you could call last minute," she said. "Fitness wasn't what I did. It was who I was."

In August 2018, a four-hundred-pound weight fell across her knees during a training session. "I lost feeling from the knees down for almost thirty minutes," she said. Refusing surgery, she trained for month while wearing a heavy knee brace, determined to heal herself. "I was determined to move," she told me. "The goal wasn't perfection. The goal was progression."

By January, she had rebuilt her strength. Days later, while flying to California for a fitness event, she noticed something strange. "My legs felt like they weighed two hundred pounds," she said. "I flipped myself upside down, with my feet where my head should have been."

Her life now is a ministry of motion. She teaches survivors to move with what they have, using socks as resistance bands, chairs for balance, and mirrors to retrain the brain. "We don't wait to be whole to move," she said. "We move to become whole."

Tracey Brown survived a stroke that should have taken her, a blood clot that should have stopped her heart, and a cancer that could have gone unnoticed. Yet here she is, lifting others as she once lifted herself.

Healing begins in the mind, transforms the body, and restores the spirit. Through faith, movement, and purpose, we don't just recover; we rise.
– Tracey Brown

Closing Reflection

Tracey's story is more than recovery. It is a revival. She reminds us that healing isn't about going back to who we were, but about becoming who we were always meant to be. Every lift, every step, every breath is both a prayer answered and a testimony in motion.

She is living proof that faith can move what medicine cannot. For Tracey Brown, healing isn't a moment. It's a mission. Her trademarked motto is *Make It a LyfeStyle™,* and we couldn't agree more. We hope her story will encourage you to find the mission that will make you better from the inside out.

Workout Tips for Post Stroke Recovery from BodyTraceFit

Survival isn't just about learning to live again. It's about learning to rise again. My scars became my testimony, proof that God can turn pain into purpose when you let faith lead the way. – Tracey Brown

Bed–Accessible Exercise: Assisted Leg Lifts

Lie on your back and use your stronger leg or hand to lift your weaker leg. Even the slightest movement reconnects the brain and body.

Chair-Accessible Exercise: Chair Marches
Sit tall with feet flat on the floor. Lift one knee, then the other. These gentle marches strengthen the hips and core and remind your brain what movement feels like.

Standing Exercise: Wall Chops
Stand with your back close to a wall. Raise both arms overhead, guiding the weaker arm with the stronger. Lower both arms as you lift one knee. Each controlled motion builds balance and hope.

Tymiak Hawkins: Guided by the Light

Taura

I came across Tymiak Hawkins's story and was instantly inspired. His strength and faith drew me in before I even knew all the details. What struck me first was his age when the stroke occurred. He was only twenty-nine, a time in life when most people think about beginnings, careers, families, and dreams just starting to take shape.

When I first learned about him, I was moved not only by what he endured but also by how he carried himself. He was playing sports, preparing to marry the love of his life, and walking with the light of possibility when everything changed. His story reminded me that every testimony has a test, and his is a living example of how faith and determination can turn the hardest trials into a message of hope.

In the weeks leading up to that day, his body had been sending signals. It began with a numbness in his foot that would not go away, a feeling he compared to a pebble stuck in his shoe. The sensation crept up his leg, making even the simplest steps feel strange. At work, the sharp focus he once relied on began to slip. He struggled with tasks that had always come easily, staring at the schedule he was supposed to finish and unable to concentrate. His boss urged him to take a break, step outside, and breathe some air. Eventually, he went home to rest, convinced that sleep would fix whatever was wrong.

The symptoms Tymiak was experiencing are common warning signs of a hemorrhagic stroke, which occurs when a weakened blood vessel ruptures, causing bleeding in or around the brain. His stroke occurred at the brain stem, a critical area that controls balance, breathing, and basic life functions. Warning signs often include numbness, dizziness, vision changes, confusion, or loss of coordination. Unlike strokes caused by clots, hemorrhagic strokes can worsen quickly because of swelling and pressure, making prompt medical care essential.

There are two main types of strokes: ischemic strokes, caused by clots that block blood flow to the brain, and hemorrhagic strokes, caused by bleeding in the brain. Both are emergencies, but hemorrhagic strokes often progress more rapidly because of swelling and pressure buildup.

The facts explain the science, but for Tymiak, those warnings were not just symptoms on a page. They were real-life moments that became harder to ignore.

On a day that should have been filled with joy, Tymiak and his now-wife, Rachel Hawkins, were preparing for his pre-wedding photos, a milestone he and his then-fiancée had been anticipating. Yet the warnings that began as whispers grew louder. His vision blurred until he could only make out colors, not details. His balance faltered, and the ground beneath him no longer felt steady. She looked closely at his face and saw something different, a subtle droop she could not ignore.

Even before the photo shoot, he was already struggling to drive. On the way to the bank, only minutes from home, he felt so off that he decided not to risk it. So, instead of driving himself to get a haircut, he ordered an Uber. Later, on the way to the photo shoot, the blurriness worsened. He recalls that he could only recognize the color of the car in front of him, not its make or any details. Still, he pressed forward, determined not to let illness steal a day that meant so much.

Rachel asked if he wanted to go to the hospital, but he brushed the concern aside. He insisted on going ahead with the photo shoot. This was supposed to be a celebration, a memory they would hold onto for the rest of their lives. He did not want sickness to intrude on such a moment. Together, they went, carrying both excitement and uncertainty into what should have been one of the happiest days of their lives.

After the photo shoot, exhaustion hit him hard. He and his fiancée went home, and he tried to eat, but after just a few bites, he felt overwhelmingly tired. He decided to lie down and rest, still hoping that sleep might help.

In the haze of sleep, something happened that he would never forget. Darkness seemed to close in around him, and in the midst of that cloud he heard a voice. "Do you trust me?" it asked. He knew instantly that it was God speaking. He answered yes. The voice responded, "Then we have to go."

He woke immediately, shook Rachel, and told her they needed to go to the hospital right away. She listened, and together they headed for the emergency room, finally yielding to the urgency his body had been signaling for weeks.

At the hospital, doctors acted quickly. He was taken for testing, and at first they believed they had found a mass. As the doctor delivered the news, Tymiak recalls seeing a figure in the corner of the room. The voice came again, reminding him, "Remember that I am going to protect you." That assurance stayed with him as the medical team worked to understand what had happened.

Further scans revealed the truth. A cavernous malformation had ruptured, causing a hemorrhagic stroke in the brain stem. The location made it especially dangerous, but he was spared surgery because his body began to reabsorb the blood naturally. He was given steroids to reduce swelling and admitted to intensive care.

Cavernous malformations are clusters of abnormal blood vessels that can sometimes appear as tumors or masses on scans. When they rupture, they may cause bleeding in the brain and can be mistaken for other conditions at first until further imaging is performed.

Road to Recovery

Tymiak spent a week in intensive care while doctors monitored him closely. He could not walk on his own and relied on a walker and the support of others to move even short distances. He was then transferred to an acute rehabilitation facility, where he spent three weeks in physical therapy, occupational therapy, and speech therapy. Every day was a test of patience and perseverance.

He remembers the small victories as clearly as the major ones. Taking a few steps down the hallway, lifting his hand, forming words more clearly, each was a sign of progress, a glimpse of the life he was fighting to reclaim. By the end of those three weeks, he was able to walk on his own again and even jog a few steps down the hall. His recovery was not complete, but it was enough to show that his determination and faith were carrying him forward.

What kept him focused was a vision. His wedding was set for three months later, and he held onto that date as his reason to keep pushing forward. He refused to accept the idea that he would need a cane or a wheelchair to walk down the aisle. Each morning, he woke up ready to work toward that vision, driven by love and supported by Rachel, his mother, and his care team.

What really stands out to me is how both my mother and Tymiak leaned on visualization, manifestation and personal goals to navigate recovery. My mother pictured herself walking the red carpet again, not in a wheelchair but standing tall in her dress. Tymiak pictured himself walking down the aisle at his wedding, strong and unassisted. Those images became their "why," the vision that gave them strength when the work of healing felt impossible. Their stories remind me that recovery is not only physical; it is also fueled by hope, purpose, and the determination to see ourselves living fully again.

Three months later, Tymiak embodied his vision. On his wedding day he walked into the wedding without assistance, a living testimony of resilience and faith.

Becoming a Light

Today, Tymiak shares his story with others so they know they are not alone. Sports will always be part of who he is. Before his stroke, he thrived on the rhythm of basketball, and even now he continues therapy to regain strength and return to the game he loves. For him, physical activity is not just exercise; it is joy, and it reminds him of the life God has preserved.

He often says that recovery never truly ends. Even years later, he still attends therapy sessions, not because he has to but because he chooses to. He works on balance through vestibular therapy, builds endurance through physical training, and sees every step forward as proof of God's grace.

Faith is now the center of his life. Each morning begins with scripture, devotionals, and quiet time to align his heart with God's plan. He no longer chases success for its own sake. Instead, he chooses purpose. He chooses gratitude. He chooses light.

Tymiak also speaks especially to men, urging them to take their health seriously, keep up with yearly checkups, and never brush off stroke warning signs. He reminds all survivors that no two recoveries are the same and that comparing yourself to others only steals joy. His advice is simple but powerful: know the signs, listen to your body, and hold on to a "why" that keeps you moving forward.

He poured these lessons into his book, *BECOMING A LIGHT*, a title that reflects both his story and his mission. It is a record of the hardest season of his life and a guide for anyone walking through their own.

Today, Tymiak embodies that light. He is a husband, a brother, an athlete, a believer, and a survivor who carries wisdom far beyond his years. His life is proof that faith can carry us through what feels impossible, that purpose can transform suffering, and that light can shine even in the darkest places.

Mindy W.: Practice Makes Purpose

I have known Mindy for more than twenty years. Long before she became a lawyer. Long before her life was shaped by briefs, deadlines, high-rise buildings, courtrooms, and the particular pressure that comes with being responsible for outcomes that affect other people's lives. The young girl and music lover that I met in the early 2000's became a class action and commercial litigation attorney. She was also my lawyer at one point, but I knew her before any of that. Before work became the center of her universe.

She has always been someone who could hold a lot at once, who could think several steps ahead, and keep going. In the years leading up to her stroke, she was working constantly. Long days, high stress, and very little rest, but as a young professional in the law field, that is kind of what you do. In my early songwriting days, I would arrive at the studio at 6 pm, maybe start writing at 8 or 9, and then record until 4-5 am on average. That's not sustainable, and certainly not my schedule now. Mindy and I had not talked in a while when she commented on a post about this book, casually mentioning that she had had a stroke too. I remember staring at my phone, rereading the sentence, trying to reconcile it with the person I knew. I was shocked. Not because I doubted her, but because I never would have imagined it happening to her. Strokes still live in our minds as something that happens to heavy, stressed-out, or older people, and Mindy's was none of those things.

It's important to note that about a month before the stroke, Mindy had forgotten the password to her computer, and she knew that was a big deal. She told a friend and the next call was to the doctor. She went in for a check-up, and they didn't find anything. Things leading up to the day of her stroke were fine, with the exception of the day before. She just felt off. She was quiet and withdrawn, and noticeably so to one of her work friends. While leaving the office for the day, her coworker told her to go home and get some rest. Another small detail is that she had a headache. Not a blaring one or the kind you panic over. Just a headache. The kind that blends into stress and easily goes away with ibuprofen. So, as most of us do when we have headaches, she just wanted to close her eyes and sleep. Sometime in the middle of the night, she woke up feeling strange. Not frightened. Not disoriented enough to tell anyone, but just off. She went to the bathroom, then back to bed. Her head still hurting, and her body felt unsettled, so she thought she might be coming down with the flu or something. Quite honestly, we've all felt this way, and unfortunately, there is no blueprint for intuition…so again, she did what we all would have done. She bundled up and went back to sleep.

The next afternoon, her phone rang. It was the same co-worker friend who told her that she should go home and get some rest. Mindy answered, believing she sounded fine, but her friend immediately realized that further action was needed. Something in her voice felt wrong. Later, the coworker would tell her she had called several times before Mindy picked up, though Mindy only remembered hearing the phone ring once.

Her coworker was alarmed that Mindy hadn't shown up for work. What happened next still feels like a quiet miracle. The coworker didn't have her emergency contacts or a direct connection to her family, but she remembered that she had helped plan Mindy's forty-fifth birthday with Mindy's sister-in-law through Facebook, and she thought maybe her number was within that thread, and it was! Mindy's sister-in-law never answers unknown calls. Ever. And as a card-carrying member of the DNA (DO NOT ANSWER) club, I know that I will not answer any call unless it has a name that I know attached to it, but something about that call felt different, so she answered.

She and Mindy's older brother were at lunch and raced to Mindy's home. Both certified nurses, trained to notice subtle changes, asked Mindy questions, but she insisted she was fine. Her sister-in-law noticed there was something wrong with Mindy's voice and continued to assess her. That's a big lesson here. If you sense something is off with a loved one, trust your instincts and keep watching them. Mindy got up to use the restroom. She was walking fine, but her sister-in-law asked her to leave the door open, just in case. Mindy reluctantly agreed, but this proved to be a life-saving request. Inside, she struggled to flush the toilet. Again and again. Watching this, her sister-in-law didn't hesitate. She knew something was very wrong, so she told Mindy's brother to call an ambulance.

After several tests at the hospital, doctors later explained that Mindy had suffered an intracranial hemorrhage of the left putamen. A hemorrhagic stroke. At the time, Mindy didn't fully grasp the magnitude of what happened. Like my mother, she learned that she had undiagnosed high blood pressure. She attributes this to being glued to her desk, eating later, and genetics. We joked about how deliciously deep-fried, smothered, and covered so many soul food and Chinese dishes are, and Mindy represents the best of both of those worlds, with a Chinese father and a black mother. Following a brief stay at the hospital, Mindy was transferred to a rehab facility and physically recovered fairly quickly, but what lingered was aphasia and dysarthria. Words didn't come as easily, and for someone whose mind had always moved fast, this was deeply frustrating, even if she didn't dwell on it out loud.

When she was discharged from the rehab facility, she stayed with her parents for a few months. It made sense. It was safe and familiar. But her doctors noticed something important. Mindy wasn't talking much. Not because she couldn't, but because she didn't have to. Her parents filled in gaps and anticipated her needs. Her doctor recommended that she return home and be around her peers. Around people who would talk with her, not for her, and would naturally draw her into conversation and help her continue rebuilding her speech. It was a turning point. She went back. Slowly, her language came back into rhythm. Conversations flowed more easily. Confidence returned. She kept going. She also lost 30 pounds and slowly started to dance with the new rhythm of life, this time with more rest, pressure limits, and lots of time spent with her brothers, sister-in-law and her niece.

Today, Mindy is back at work and doing extremely well. She is sharp. Engaged and still herself, but now with boundaries and goals beyond the desk. She beat the odds, just like every survivor in this book. Her story stays with me not because of how dramatic it was, but because of how close it lived to *normal*. How easily it could have gone another way and how terribly sad I would have been if it did.

Another huge takeaway is how much her survival depended on people paying attention when she could not. May this be a reminder to be intentional about who you surround yourself with, even at work.

I am so proud of Mindy and her resilience, but honestly, if someone was going to fight like hell to come out standing tall on the other side, it would be her.

When we first spoke, she was traveling back from a law convention, just like the Mindy that I know so well. Always learning and growing. She's always done that for her clients, but now she is doing it for herself, too.

CHAPTER SIX

SURVIVORS HANDBOOK

Yvonne

So much was covered in the Caregiver's Handbook, but I also want to hold space for us, the survivors. If you have survived a stroke, congratulations. As I have said before, get moving. I do not care if it is just your eyes, move them back and forth. Climb the mountain in your mind and jump into the river below. It all starts in your mind.

Here are some other tips that will be helpful to you:

- Start small, but start: Every movement counts. Wiggle your toes, stretch your fingers, and turn your head. The body follows where the mind leads.

- Keep a routine: Recovery thrives on rhythm. Take your medications on time, show up for therapy, and track your progress.

- Celebrate small victories: Every step, every word, and every meal prepared is a win. Do not overlook your progress.

- Protect your peace: Avoid toxic environments and surround yourself with encouragement. Stress weighs on the body more than we realize.

- Nourish your body: Eat foods that support healing, drink water, and rest when your body asks for it.

- Stay connected: Isolation slows healing. Stay engaged with family, friends, or a support group.

- Use your voice: Tell people what you need. Advocate for yourself in appointments and in daily life.

- Keep learning: Challenge your brain with puzzles, music, journaling, or prayer. The brain is always capable of healing and growing.

- Never ignore warning signs: If you experience new or recurring symptoms, seek medical attention right away.

What to Expect on the Journey

Recovery after a stroke is rarely simple or predictable. Healing can progress, pause, and sometimes feel like it is moving backward. Knowing what to expect can help you stay encouraged and patient with yourself.

- **Sundowning and speech changes**: Many survivors notice that speech may improve at times, and then become more difficult again, especially later in the day. This is often called sundowning and is usually tied to fatigue. It does not mean you are losing progress. Recovery often comes in waves rather than in a straight line.

- **Physical setbacks**: Muscles can feel stronger one day and weaker the next. Balance and coordination may also fluctuate. Keep moving, even if progress feels uneven, but be very careful with activities like cooking, cleaning, driving, or other tasks that could hurt you or others.

- **Emotional shifts**: Mood swings, irritability, or unexpected sadness may appear. This is not a sign of weakness; it is the brain adjusting. Support from loved ones, counseling, or support groups can make a big difference.

- **Memory challenges**: Short-term memory and focus may take time to rebuild. Notes, reminders, and repetition can help you stay on track as your brain heals.

Giving Yourself Time

One of the most important lessons I have learned on this journey is to give yourself time. I am naturally more introspective, while my daughter likes to talk things through. Add to that the stress of being in an unfamiliar city, and the weight of recovery can put strain on relationships. A stroke changes everything, including routines, roles, and even the way you communicate. It is easy to grow frustrated with yourself and with the people closest to you.

What helped me, and what I hope will help you, is to remember that healing takes time and that caring for your mental health is just as vital as caring for your physical health.

Here are some ways to support yourself:

- **Commit to talking with a therapist**: My mom and I went to therapy , and it was helpful, but I also recommend scheduling time to speak with a therapist on your own. Both shared and private sessions can give you space to process feelings in different ways.

- **TRY WRITTEN OR AUDIBLE JOURNALING**: Writing down thoughts, fears, or victories can help release emotions that are hard to say out loud. It also helps track progress you might not notice day by day. If you are unable to write anything down just yet, record your journal entries using your phone's voice note feature.

- **Practice mindfulness or meditation**: A few minutes of quiet breathing, prayer, or stillness can calm the nervous system and restore focus.

- **Stay open with loved ones**: Share when you feel tired, sad, or overwhelmed rather than keeping it inside. Clear communication prevents misunderstandings and helps others know how to support you.

- **Allow rest without guilt**: Healing is work. If you need to step back from social events or daily routines to protect your energy, give yourself permission to do so.

- **Join a support group**: Whether online or in person, connecting with others who understand the stroke journey can be comforting and encouraging.

Commit to the Work

Therapy may not be something you are interested in, but I encourage you to commit to it. At first, you or your loved one might resist the idea, but I am sure that you will find it to be one of the most important parts of   your healing. Talking with a professional gives us new tools, a fresh perspective, and a place to speak freely without fear of burdening family. It may not be easy, but it will be worth it.

I also encourage you to return to the Caregiver's Handbook. Read it not only for information but also to understand what your loved ones may be carrying. Seeing their side of the journey can help you meet each other with more patience and compassion.

Other practices that support recovery include:

- **Faith and prayer**: Leaning into spiritual practices and places of worship can bring peace and strength in difficult moments.
- **Creative expression**: Painting, singing, cooking, or writing poems can unlock joy and release emotions that may be hard to put into words.
- **Gentle movement**: Chair exercises, stretching, or walking short distances can build strength and confidence.
- **Education**: Learn as much as you can about stroke and your own health. Knowledge is power and can guide the decisions you make every day.
- **Celebrating victories**: Keep a record of milestones, no matter how small, and revisit them when you need encouragement.

AUTONOMOUS PHYSICAL THERAPY

Before I share these, let me remind you again to always check with your doctor before starting any exercise, even small ones. Every stroke is different, and your medical team knows what is safe for you. My second reminder is about consistency. Improvement comes from doing a little each day. Progress may feel slow at times, but showing up daily makes all the difference.

There are some exercises that helped my mom with recovery that she did right at home:

For hands and fingers

- Stretch your fingers wide, then slowly bring them together to make a fist. Repeat several times.
- Touch each fingertip to your thumb, one at a time, as if you were playing an invisible piano.
- Place a soft ball or a rolled-up sock in your hand and squeeze gently, then release.
- Practice opening and closing clothespins or snapping buttons to build strength.
- Roll a small ball back and forth on the table under your palm to wake up the nerves.

For arms and shoulders

- Sit tall and slowly raise your arms above your head, then lower them. If needed, guide the weaker arm with the stronger one.
- Shrug your shoulders toward your ears, hold for a few seconds, then relax.
- Make gentle circles with your arms, forward and backward, as if swimming.
- Use a towel or scarf: hold it with both hands and raise it overhead, then lower it.

For legs and feet

- While sitting, march your legs in place, lifting one knee at a time.
- Flex and point your toes several times to keep your ankles flexible.
- Stand near a counter or sturdy chair and practice shifting your weight from one leg to the other.
- Heel-to-toe walk across a safe surface to improve balance.
- Sit and extend one leg straight, hold for a moment, then lower it slowly.

For speech and voice

- Read aloud, even if only a few sentences at a time.
- Practice tongue twisters slowly and clearly.
- Follow along with voice therapy videos on YouTube and repeat the exercises daily.
- Sing your favorite song, starting with humming if forming words is hard.
- Exaggerate mouth movements by pronouncing vowels (A, E, I, O, U) slowly and clearly.

For facial movement

- Practice big smiles: even if one side does not move fully, keep trying. Hold for a few seconds, then relax.
- Raise your eyebrows as high as you can, then lower them. Repeat several times.
- Pucker your lips as if you are going to whistle or blow a kiss, then relax.
- Alternate between saying "ooo" and "eee" slowly and clearly, exaggerating the lip shapes.
- Try gentle cheek puffs: fill your mouth with air and push it from one cheek to the other. If air escapes on one side, gently use your hand to support your lips until they grow stronger.
- Use a mirror so you can see both sides of your face. Watching yourself helps the brain reconnect to those muscles.
- Massage the weaker side of your face with clean hands, using small circles to stimulate awareness.

For neck strength and flexibility

- Sit up straight and slowly turn your head to the right, then back to center, then to the left. Move gently and only as far as is comfortable.
- Tilt your head so your right ear moves toward your right shoulder, then back to center, then to the left. Keep your shoulders relaxed.

- Gently nod your head forward as if saying yes, then lift your chin toward the ceiling.
- Slowly shake your head as if saying no, moving side to side in a controlled way.
- Try small neck circles, rolling your head slowly forward, to the side, back, and around.
- Place your hand lightly on your forehead, then push your head forward into your hand without moving your neck. Hold for a few seconds, then relax. Do the same with your hand on the back of your head and on each side to build strength.

Always move slowly and stop if you feel pain or dizziness. These gentle stretches keep the neck flexible, improve circulation, and support better posture, making breathing, speaking, and swallowing easier.

For the mind

- Do puzzles, word searches, or crosswords to strengthen focus.
- Listen to music and try singing along, even softly.
- Write down three things you are grateful for each day.
- Play simple card or matching games to sharpen your memory.
- Try memorizing short poems, scriptures, or affirmations and repeat them daily.

Each of these exercises may feel small, but small things build strength. Be gentle with yourself and stay consistent. Over time, you will see that these simple daily practices lead to real progress.

Devices and Discoveries

When I first began my healing journey, one of my favorite tools was the Medi Massager that Taura bought for me at Costco. It became my go-to for improving circulation in my legs and feet. Having something simple to use at home gave me both comfort and confidence.

There are   devices and practices that some survivors have found helpful. Not everything will be right for everyone, and it is always best to check with your doctor before starting something new. Here are a few options to consider:

Circulation and movement

- **Foot and leg massagers:** Similar to the Medi Massager, these can improve blood flow, ease stiffness, and provide comfort when walking is difficult.
- **Resistance bands:** Light bands can help rebuild strength in arms and legs through gentle, guided exercises.
- **Hand therapy balls:** Squeezing soft balls or therapy putty can help improve grip and finger strength.
- **Lymphatic drainage massage:** Gentle self-massage or professional lymphatic drainage can reduce swelling, improve circulation, and help the body clear toxins. This can be as simple as lightly brushing the skin toward the heart with your hands or using a soft, dry brush.

Advanced therapies

- **Hyperbaric oxygen chambers**: These deliver oxygen under pressure, and some studies suggest they may help the brain recover by improving oxygen delivery. Results vary, so it is important to discuss this with a medical professional.
- **Red light therapy**: Low-level light applied to the body may support circulation and tissue healing. It is still being studied, but many people find it soothing.

Relaxation and support

- **Weighted blankets:** These can help calm the nervous system, improve sleep, and reduce anxiety.
- **Heating pads and cold packs:** Alternating heat and cold can relax stiff muscles or ease swelling.
- **Compression socks:** These can support circulation and reduce leg swelling.

Do not overlook your insurance benefits:
Many people are unaware that their health insurance may already cover helpful services. Check your plan for benefits such as:

- **Gym memberships:** Some plans include free or discounted access to fitness centers or wellness programs.
- **Monthly massages:** Massage therapy may be covered when prescribed by a doctor and can improve circulation, reduce stress, and ease muscle tension.
- **Acupuncture or chiropractic care:** These may be included under certain plans and can support pain relief and mobility.
- **Nutritionist:** A plan   designed by a dietitian may be covered and can help guide food choices that lower stroke risk.
- **Transportation services:** Some plans provide rides to medical appointments.

What we've learned is that recovery is not only about the big steps. Small tools, consistent practices, and even the hidden resources already available to you can make the daily road smoother. Explore what works for you, always with safety in mind, and give yourself permission to use the devices and benefits that bring comfort and relief.

Everyday Life After Stroke

Recovery is not only about therapy and medication. It is also about finding your way back into everyday life. Simple tasks can feel new again, and it can be frustrating when they take more time or effort, but be patient. Small adjustments can bring big relief. Here are some areas where my mom learned to adapt.

Eating and Cooking

- If swallowing is difficult, work with a speech therapist to determine safe food textures and practice swallowing exercises.
- Use adaptive utensils with larger grips if holding silverware is difficult.
- When cooking, place a non-slip mat under cutting boards and bowls.

- Try one-handed kitchen tools, such as rocker knives or jar openers.

Getting Around

- Ask your doctor or therapist about safe driving. Some survivors return to driving, while others rely on transportation services or rides from family.
- Many communities offer low-cost ride programs through insurance, senior centers, or local transit.
- If walking is hard, use a cane or walker with pride. These are tools for independence, not signs of weakness.

Managing Fatigue

- Plan your most important activities for the time of day when you have the most energy.
- Take short naps or rest breaks rather than pushing through exhaustion.
- Listen to your body. Fatigue is not failure; it is part of recovery.

Returning to Work or Hobbies

- Speak with your doctor about the type of work you can safely do and ask about vocational rehabilitation programs.
- If you cannot return to your old job right away, consider part-time work, volunteering, or hobbies that bring you joy.
- Try adapting old hobbies to your abilities. My mom baked her famous cupcakes for friends, ofen taking them to hospitals or care centers to brighten their day.

Personal Care

- **Hair:** Combing your hair can be tiring, especially with one hand. Protective styles such as braids, twists, or locs can save time and energy while keeping your hair healthy. If possible, connect with barbers or stylists who offer home visits. Avoid harsh chemicals that may irritate your scalp or require long salon visits. Gentle, natural products are often easier to manage. On days when full styling is too much, use wide-tooth combs, detangling brushes, or soft headwraps.

- **Teeth and gums:** Brushing and flossing may feel harder, but oral health is critical for stroke survivors. Use an electric toothbrush for easier brushing, and consider floss picks or water flossers if traditional flossing is difficult. Good dental care lowers inflammation and supports overall brain and heart health.

- **Bathing:** Shower chairs, grab bars, and handheld showerheads can make bathing safer and less tiring. Non-slip mats help prevent falls. DO NOT RUSH. Move slowly, and if needed, ask for help. Cleanliness not only prevents infections but also lifts your mood and builds your confidence.

- **Dressing and clothing:** Getting dressed can be challenging, but the right choices make it easier. Look for clothing with Velcro or magnetic closures instead of buttons or zippers. Slip-on shoes or those with elastic can save energy and frustration. Lay out your clothes the night before to make mornings smoother. Choose soft fabrics and loose fits on days when movement feels limited. There are also adaptive clothing lines designed specifically for people with limited mobility. Remember, comfort and independence are more important than fashion trends.

Communication and Connection

- If speech is affected, keep practicing with loved ones, using therapy apps, or by reading aloud.

- Use notebooks, phone apps, or flashcards to help when words are slow to come.

- Stay socially connected. Isolation can slow healing, while laughter and conversation can lift your spirits.

Stroke's changes how we live, but if you have been blessed with the gift of again, then rip it open and put it on!

The Dangers of Being Sedentary

One of the greatest threats after a stroke is becoming sedentary. At first, it feels natural. You are tired, your body aches, and even simple movements take so much effort. Sitting still or lying down feels safer. But staying still for too long creates a cycle that makes recovery harder. Muscles weaken, circulation slows, and the risk of another stroke or blood clot increases.

I want you to hear me clearly: rest is necessary, but a sedentary lifestyle is dangerous. Healing requires movement, even if it is the smallest step you can take today.

Why is being sedentary harmful to recovery?

- Muscles lose strength quickly when they are not used, making it harder to walk, lift, or maintain balance.
- Blood flow slows, increasing the risk of clots and swelling.
- Joints stiffen and can become painful.
- Energy levels drop, and fatigue worsens rather than improves.
- The brain receives less stimulation, which can slow its ability to rewire and heal.

Ways to break the sedentary cycle

- **Start small**: If all you can do today is lift your arm or move your eyes back and forth, that still matters. Small movements add up.
- **Set reminders**: Use a timer or an alarm to remind yourself to move every hour. Even standing for a few minutes or stretching in a chair can help.
- **Move in your chair**: March your legs while sitting, roll your shoulders, or stretch your fingers. Movement does not have to mean walking across the room.
- **Celebrate activity**: Every time you choose to move, you are investing in your recovery. Write it down or tell someone so you remember the progress you are making.
- **Get support**: Ask a loved one or caregiver to walk with you, stretch with you, or remind you when you need encouragement.

A new definition of movement
Movement is not only about exercise in the gym. Movement is

washing dishes, combing your hair, reading aloud, or standing at the window and stretching your arms. Movement is choosing to live.

Do not let the chair or the bed become your prison. Every time you move, you reclaim a little more of your life.

Resources for Survivors

These resources are designed to support you on your journey. Every stroke is different, so not all resources will meet your needs. Explore what feels right, and always talk with your doctor before starting new therapies or programs.

National Organizations

- **American Stroke Association**
  Education, advocacy, survivor stories, and community programs.
- **National Institute of Neurological Disorders and Stroke (NINDS) –**
  Research-based information on stroke types, treatments, and recovery.

Support and Community

- **Stroke support groups** – Check with your local hospital or rehabilitation center, or search Meetup's for in-person and online groups.
- **Facebook groups for stroke survivors** – Many private groups offer daily encouragement, tips, and connection.
- **National Aphasia Association** – www.aphasia.org
  Resources and support for survivors experiencing speech or language changes.

Therapy and Recovery Tools

- **Speech therapy apps** such as CONSTANT THERAPY or TACTUS THERAPY for daily home exercises.
- **OT/PT home programs** – Ask your therapist for apps or handouts to keep exercises going between visits.

- **Mindfulness and relaxation apps** such as HEADSPACE or CALM to support focus, rest, and stress relief.

As previously mentioned, some platforms do not allow external websites, so please research the following.

Mental Health and Wellness

- **Psychology Today** insurance and specialty.
- **NAMI (National Alliance on Mental Illness)**
- **Support groups for caregivers and families** – often listed through hospitals, churches, or community centers.

Financial Resources

- **BenefitsCheckUp**
- **Patient Advocate Foundation**
- **NeedyMeds**
- **Partnership for Prescription Assistance**
- **Medicare/Medicaid Extra Help Program**
- **State Vocational Rehabilitation**.
- **Hospital financial counselors**

Lifestyle and Prevention

- **Silver Sneakers**
- **YMCA Stroke Wellness Programs**

In Closing

You are a survivor, not a victim. Speak those words to yourself, daily.

And like I said before, keep moving. Movement is healing. It may be slow or small, but it is still progress. Still forward. So keep going, because every step, every thought, and every prayer is bringing you closer to the life you are meant to live.

CHAPTER SEVEN

EXPERT ADVICE

Dr. Swati Laroia Coon: The.Stroke.Doc

I first met Dr. Swati Laroia Coon the way many people do these days. I slid into her DMs. I reached out after a fruitless, endless scroll late one night that serendipitously led me to her Instagram feed, @The. Stroke.Doc. Suddenly, things felt different, inspiring even. The information felt like it was coming from someone who truly cares about humanity, or me personally, if I'm being honest. Her message didn't sound like a lecture. It sounded like a woman reaching through h the screen, saying, *THIS MESSAGE IS FOR ONE IN FOR OF YOU... MORE ON FOUR LATER.*

Known as *The Stroke Doc*, Dr. Swati Laroia Coon is a vascular neurologist and tele-neurology specialist who uses her voice to make stroke awareness practical and personal. She bridges the gap between the hospital and the home, meeting people where they are and reminding us that awareness is only powerful when paired with preparation and action.

When we spoke, she had just finished a hospital shift but made time to talk to me with full presence, as if this conversation were as important as any case. Her tone was steady, her compassion alive in every word. One of the biggest takeaways was when she said, "One in four people will have a stroke in their lifetime," she said. "Think of you and your three closest friends. One of you will be affected. The 4 number stayed with me long after our talk. I kept thinking about my three closest friends, and how easily one statistic could become a personal tragedy. Since that conversation, I have been quietly encouraging the people closest to me to take action. We trade recipes and some of us even share daily steps, but now there is a bit more intention locked behind it…4. I hope Dr. Swati's statement encourages you to lock-in on your four, you and three others and commit to make lasting changes. If we collectively set our intentions on prevention, we can beat the odds stacked against us.

Dr. Swati's view of prevention centers on overall well-being, but at the top of the wellness chain is brain health. "We talk about heart health all the time," she said, "but our brain drives everything we are. It's your personality, your memories, your movement, your voice. We should be as protective of our brains as we are of our hearts." She also spoke of good rest as brain medicine, along with other brain health suggestions we have outlined below, but one of the most beautiful things she said is:

"Blood flow is the language of life. When it slows, the body forgets its rhythm." – The Stroke Doc

Be honest. When was the last time you thought about your brain health? I'll wait… one, two, yeah… me neither. But we hope that reading Dr. Swati's passage will change that. She went on to discuss the importance of brainstem function.

"The brain and the heart share blood vessels, but the brainstem is the bridge between them. It tells the heart when to beat and the lungs when to breathe. When the brainstem is injured, those automatic systems are the first to fail," she said.

She wants readers to know that warning signs of brainstem trouble can be subtle but serious. These include sudden dizziness, imbalance, double vision, slurred speech, or difficulty swallowing. These symptoms can easily be mistaken for fatigue or vertigo, but they often indicate that the body's control center is under distress.

"The brainstem is small, but it holds everything that keeps us alive," Dr. Swati explained. "It's what connects the brain to the body. When it's affected, you don't just lose balance, you lose breath, heartbeat, rhythm."

So how do we keep our brains, hearts, and bodies healthy? Dr. Swati believes in the power of small, consistent choices. The way we move, eat, and breathe each day becomes the soil in which a long life can grow. She recommends the Mediterranean approach to eating, which I'll outline below. In short, it's about choosing foods that are nutrient-dense and life-giving. "It's not about perfection," she told me. "It's about eating to live."

Our conversation deepened when I shared my mother's story. As you may already know, before the stroke, my mother was exhausted. She drew a bath, alone in the house, hoping to rest. She heard a pop in her head and fell asleep. By the grace of God, she woke up to another chance at life, which is why this book is called The Gift of Again. When we lose loved ones, we always wish to hold them again, hear their voices again, and say I love you again. That's why "again" is such a gift. One I don't take for granted, especially after Dr. Swati warned, "Never go to sleep with stroke symptoms…don't wait to see if it passes. Call 911. Get scanned." She paused for a moment. "And please, don't reach for baby aspirin unless your doctor has prescribed it. If it's a brain bleed, you could be thinning your blood at the worst possible time."

There was something powerful about the way she said it, spoken by a woman who's seen too many stories that didn't end like my mother's. She told me again, softly but firmly, "Silence never saved a life." If you know what bars are, you know "Silence never saved a life" is a total bar. I will never forget that quote, and I hope you don't either. So here it is again.

"Silence never saved a life" – Dr. Swati

We also talked about my mom's TIA, which she had within 24-hours of the stroke. Some people call it a mini stroke, but she explained that there is no such thing as a "mini stroke." "A TIA isn't small," she said.

"It's a warning. If symptoms fade, that doesn't mean it's gone. The risk of a full stroke rises sharply in the next few days." She wanted people to understand that the body's first signal is incredibly important, but if you google "stroke symptoms," you may think you are okay if you don't have the typical symptoms. Below are other signs that Dr. Swati would like for us to familiarize ourselves with.

Uncommon stroke signs

- Sudden nausea or vomiting with no clear cause
- Heaviness in one or both legs
- Sudden loss of balance or coordination
- Difficulty swallowing or unexpected hiccups
- Sudden confusion, severe fatigue, or a fog that feels unfamiliar
- Sudden severe headache
- Popping sound in the head (added in honor of my mother's experience)

She said these symptoms often lead people to rest instead of act. To take a nap instead of a scan. To wait it out because they don't want to "overreact." But the truth is, it's better to be wrong about your stroke symptoms at a hospital than at home.

As she spoke, I thought again of my mother, how easily she could have been a story told in the past tense. I felt gratitude and responsibility settle in my chest. Gratitude that she was spared. Responsibility to share what I now know.

Dr. Swati teaches that time is brain. Every minute without oxygen kills millions of neurons, yet she delivers this truth as a promise rather than a punishment. "If you feel off, don't wait for morning," she said. "Call now."

We started our conversation with her asking herself what if she could put a yard sign on everyone's lawn, about stroke prevention and awareness. Since she can't, social media has been her virtual yard sign. The sign is simple and direct. It says:

Know the Signs. Save a Life!

Other things that   I have learned from The.Stroke.Docs proverbial yard sign is that health isn't found in extremes but in the quiet consistency of care. She says,

"As a society, we invest heavily in looking younger on the outside, yet the real key to aging gracefully lies in nurturing our bodies and minds from within, prioritizing brain and body health over quick cosmetic fixes." – Dr. Swati

That landed heavily on me as a resident of Los Angeles, the land of perfection. We stretch, smooth, and sculpt our reflections, chasing youth as if it were proof of life. But maybe the fountain of youth lives beneath the surface. Maybe it's in the quiet work of keeping your mind clear, your blood flowing, and your spirit at rest. For me and my mom, and many of you, it's in prayer and faith. When your health is compromised, you learn quickly that getting it back is all that matters. The mirror doesn't mean as much when you're lying in bed, looking back on your life. What matters then is how you cared for the body that carried you, the mind that held your memories, and the faith that kept you here. Maybe real beauty is being righteous to ourselves and our neighbors, treating both the body we live in and the people we live beside with great kindness and respect, and letting our voices be louder than fear.

I am so incredibly inspired to do better after my conversation with The Stroke Doc, and I hope you are too. This has been an eye-opening lesson, and below I've recapped some of the most important things to remember, along with a few extra gems the good Stroke Doc shared. I'm deeply grateful for this exchange with such an extraordinary human, and I encourage you to find her on social media or whatever emerging technology comes next. Just look for the doctor with glowing skin, a healthy brain, and the biggest heart.

Brain Health Tips from The Stroke Doc

- Get consistent, quality sleep. It allows the brain to clear toxins and reset.

- Drink water throughout the day. Dehydration thickens the blood and slows circulation.

- Move your body daily. Even gentle stretching or walking improves circulation and oxygen flow.

- Eat for circulation. Choose foods that nourish rather than numb.

- Keep stress low. Chronic stress constricts blood vessels and clouds the mind.

- Check your blood pressure regularly. Know your numbers before an emergency does.

- Stay connected. Conversation, laughter, and community protect mental health.

- Challenge your mind. Read, write, sing, pray, or learn something new.

- Listen to your body. Sudden fatigue, dizziness, or imbalance are not small matters.

- Protect your heart to protect your brain. They share the same vessels and the same story.

Stroke Prevention Basics

- Recognize that awareness saves lives. The faster you act, the more brain you save.

- Know the signs. Not just the common ones, but the subtle ones, too.

- Never go to sleep on new symptoms or take a bath if you feel "off."

- Call 911. Do not wait to see if it passes.

- Do not take aspirin unless your own doctor has prescribed it.

- Keep blood pressure, cholesterol, and stress within healthy ranges.

- Schedule yearly checkups and ask your doctor about your risk factors.

- Move more, smoke less, rest deeply, and eat foods that keep blood flowing freely.

- Remember that silence never saved a life. Speak up. Act quickly. Trust your body.

The Mediterranean and Mind *Livit*

I've never liked the word diet. It says DIE-T, and I take that quite personally, ha. So, let's call this a *livit* instead, a way of living that feeds the body and the soul.

As mentioned earlier, Dr. Swati recommends the Mediterranean approach to eating and the Dash Diet (*Livit*) to control salt intake. She says excess salt in our diets increases our risk of hypertension, which is also known as the silent killer and can lead to strokes and heart disease. There are many books and blogs that explore both of these protocols in detail, but the list below will help you get started.

The Basics of the Mediterranean *Livit*

- Eat mostly plants, vegetables, fruits, beans, and whole grains.
- Choose healthy fats like olive oil, nuts, and seeds.
- Enjoy fish and seafood a few times a week for protein and omega-3s.
- Limit red meat and processed foods; make them occasional, not daily.
- Season with herbs and gratitude instead of salt.
- Drink water often and wine sparingly, if at all.
- Share meals when you can; conversation and community are part of nourishment.
- Move your body after eating; even a short walk helps circulation.
- Rest well. The brain cleans itself while you sleep.
- Give thanks for what's on your plate and for who's beside you.

DASH Nutrition Protocol

- Begin each day with plenty of water
- Fill half the plate with vegetables or fruit at every meal
- Choose whole grains such as brown rice, quinoa, oats, and whole-grain bread
- Use lean proteins, including fish, poultry, tofu, and beans

- Include low-fat or fat-free dairy for calcium and added protein
- Add nuts and seeds in small portions a few times a week
- Cook with healthy oils like olive oil
- Limit sodium by choosing fresh foods and reading labels for lower-salt options
- Season with herbs, citrus, garlic, or spices in place of salt
- Reduce intake of foods high in sugar, including sweets, sugary drinks, and refined snacks
- Keep red meat and processed meats to occasional meals
- Aim for high fiber choices to support heart health and digestion
- Prepare meals at home as often as possible to maintain consistency
- Support the protocol with regular movement and mindful habits

Jerome Lawrence: From Oakland to Holistic Healing

We first met Jerome Lawrence when he was a teenager, and Taura was still a little girl. I was a hairstylist then, churning out press-and-curl and Jheri curls, first from my kitchen and later from my basement. At the time, Jerome was working at McDonald's with his friend Arlester Washington, who also became like family to us. Both Jerome and Arlester had a barter system with me. They would bring us food from the Golden Arches in exchange for a bouncy Jheri curl. Yes, it was the 80s, and they used to say my curls were bangin'…the best in the west.

Back on a more serious note, Jerome's life was not all golden back then. It was fast and dangerous. We didn't see him in the drive-thru that much anymore, and now he and many of my clients pulled up in fancy cars with music that rattled my entire house. Oakland in the crack era was not an easy place for young men, and like many others, he was caught between fast money and slow change. So many guys I knew, either my clients or the boyfriends of my clients, ended up dead or in jail, but this is not one of those stories. Jerome's story is still being written, and my God, is it beautiful! To see him now is to see a completely different man. He has chosen healing over hustle, wisdom over impulse, and a healthy path instead of one riddled with fast food and faster living.

Jerome's turning point came through his mother's health struggles. She suffered two strokes and a heart attack, and though she has since passed, her journey became the reason he dedicated himself to holistic medicine. What began as a son trying to help his mother has grown into a purpose that now touches countless lives.

Jerome is a walking testament to change. His deep knowledge of nutrition and plant medicine is rooted in both science and ancestral wisdom, and his Zenny water and herbs are restoring health for many in the Bay Area and beyond. When Jerome speaks about stress, diet, and the toll of trauma, he speaks as both a teacher and a survivor, someone who has lived on both sides of sickness and healing.

Stress and Trauma

Jerome believes many strokes in the Black community begin with stress. He explains that trauma can be passed down through generations and still affect us today. Witnessing injustice can trigger the same physical and emotional responses our grandparents felt, keeping the body in fight-or-flight for too long.

He says, "Stress might not always look like what we think it does. It can hide in our habits, our silence, even our strength." Science supports what Jerome feels in his spirit. According to the *JOURNAL OF THE AMERICAN HEART ASSOCIATION*, people living under constant stress are more than twice as likely to experience a stroke. In a global study published in *JAMA NETWORK OPEN*, which followed more than twenty-six thousand people, those who reported high stress at home or at work were nearly two to three times more likely to have a stroke. The same study found that psychological distress alone increased the likelihood of stroke by one hundred seventeen percent, even when age, weight, and blood pressure were taken into account.

For women, the connection is especially strong. A 2025 study published in *NEUROLOGY* found that women under fifty who reported moderate stress had a seventy-eight percent higher risk of stroke, and that risk rose with higher stress levels. Another review published in *FRONTIERS IN NEUROLOGY* found that veterans and others living with post-traumatic stress disorder faced a fifty-nine percent higher risk of stroke. The evidence is clear. Chronic stress puts pressure on the body that builds silently over time, tightening vessels, raising blood pressure, and wearing the heart down.

Still, Jerome insists there is hope. He believes that what we put into our minds and spirits each day can shape our health as much as what we eat or drink.

His remedy:

- **Begin each day with prayer or meditation** to calm the mind and settle the body. A peaceful start can lower blood pressure and prepare the heart to handle whatever comes.

- **Practice breathing and stillness** to shift into healing mode. Even five minutes of slow, deep breathing can reset the nervous system and quiet racing thoughts.

- **Create safe outlets for stress, especially for Black men** who often carry their pain alone. Talk to someone you trust, move your body, write, or pray. Do not hold it all inside.

- **Protect your peace daily.** Turn off the news when it becomes too heavy. Spend time in nature. Laugh often. Feed your spirit as much as you feed your body.

Stress and Stroke by Numbers

- **2x** — People living with chronic stress are more than twice as likely to experience a stroke

- **2 to 3x** — Those who report high stress at home or at work are nearly two to three times as likely to suffer a stroke as those who do not.

- **117%** — Psychological distress, such as chronic anxiety or a sense of powerlessness, increases the risk of stroke by more than one hundred percent, even after adjusting for blood pressure and age.

- **78%** — Women under fifty who live with moderate stress have a seventy-eight percent higher risk of stroke.

- **59%** —Veterans and others living with post-traumatic stress disorder face a nearly sixty percent higher risk.
- **1 in 6** — According to the World Stroke Organization's PREVENT STROKE campaign, about one in six strokes worldwide is linked to stress or depression.

We agree with Jerome, who poignantly says:

"Peace is not a luxury. It is protection." – Jerome Lawrence

The more we honor our need for rest and stillness, the more we give our bodies a fighting chance to heal.

Diet and Digestion

Food is medicine, but Jerome warns that processed foods and sugar stripped of fiber overwhelm the liver and lead to plaque buildup in the arteries.

His remedy:

- Add fiber to every meal, especially inulin, a plant fiber that can be sprinkled over food or blended into smoothies
- Eat dark, leafy greens and colorful fruits every day
- Swap some animal protein for plant-based options and sea vegetables, which support heart health without producing plaque

Emotional and Spiritual Health

Jerome reminds us that unspoken pain is just as damaging as poor nutrition. He says men, especially, need spaces where they can release what they carry instead of holding it in silence.

His remedy:

- Create spaces for vulnerability and openness
- Choose connection and community over isolation

- Practice prayer, meditation, or reflection daily

Menopause and Cholesterol

Jerome teaches that the drop in estrogen during menopause makes women more vulnerable to stroke because the liver can no longer regulate cholesterol. Doesn't that make so much sense?

His remedy:

- Support hormone health with plant-based foods, omega-3s, magnesium, and vitamin D
- Avoid processed dairy and cheese, which unnaturally raise estrogen levels
- Pay close attention to triglyceride and HDL levels in blood work

To Supplement or Not to Supplement?

Jerome teaches that most of us cannot rely on food alone to protect our health because food today is not what it used to be. The soil has been depleted, crops are harvested too early, and much of what reaches our plates has lost the minerals and vitality our grandparents once counted on. "You can eat a tomato today and it doesn't have the same vitamins and minerals as the tomato your grandmother grew in her yard," Jerome explains. "That's why we need supplements. Food just isn't what it used to be."

Supplements, in his view, do not replace food; they are food's greatest helper! They work alongside what we eat to restore what has been stripped away. When we add magnesium, omega-3s, vitamin C, or beetroot, we are not bypassing food but strengthening it, giving our meals back the power they once naturally held.

Voices that Echo Jerome

Listening to Jerome reminded us that he is not alone in his approach. Many respected holistic doctors and practitioners have been teaching the same truths in their own ways.

- **Queen Afua**, author of *SACRED WOMAN*, teaches that detoxifying the body with live, plant-based foods, herbs, and spiritual practices is essential to Black wellness and generational healing.

- **Dr. Sebi** believed that hybridized and processed foods lack the minerals necessary for true cellular health, and he taught that natural plants, herbs, and mineral-rich water are the foundation of healing.

- **Dr. Mark Hyman** is a functional medicine pioneer who emphasizes that food is medicine and links chronic disease to processed diets and nutrient-depleted soil.

- **Dr. Andrew Weil** advocates anti-inflammatory diets rich in fiber, omega-3s, and plant-based nutrients, recognizing inflammation as the root of many modern illnesses, including heart disease and strokes.

- **Dr. Joel Fuhrman** is known for his "nutritarian" diet, which emphasizes the importance of micronutrient-dense foods such as leafy greens, beans, and fruits to prevent disease and extend life.

- **Dr. Dean Ornish** demonstrated through clinical studies that plant-based eating, stress reduction, and lifestyle changes can reverse heart disease and lower stroke risk.

- **Dr. Joseph Mercola** warns about soil depletion and food quality, encouraging supplementation with magnesium, vitamin D, and omega 3s as essential for long-term health.

Together, these voices echo Jerome's journey. They affirm that true healing begins when we see food as medicine, honor plants, minerals, and herbs as tools of restoration, and take seriously our responsibility to give our bodies back what the modern world has stripped away.

Jerome's essentials:

- Omega-3s to calm inflammation and keep the heart strong
- Vitamin C to cleanse blood vessels and strengthen immunity
- Magnesium to relax arteries and improve circulation
- Beetroot and other nitric oxide boosters to open blood vessels and lower pressure

- Combination blends, like his "Rebirth" formula, that bring these nutrients together in harmony

In Jerome's words,

"Supplements don't replace food; they complete it. They give the body back what the modern world has taken away."

Jessica Brewer, Physician Associate–Certified

Functional and metabolic medicine specialist restoring balance from root causes.

When I think of Jessica Brewer, the word that comes to mind is lifeline. I came to her at a period when I felt stuck. I was eating right, exercising, and doing everything I thought I was supposed to, but my body was not responding. The scale would not budge, my energy was low, and I felt like I was losing the fight with my own health.

Another provider had put me on GLP-1 medication, but instead of it helping, it left me feeling sick and drained. I knew that could not be the only option. I wanted to feel better, not worse. Jessica stepped in and changed everything. She helped me see that health is not only about calories or exercise; it is about balance. She started with my digestion, because if your gut is out of order, nothing else can fall into place. From there, she opened up a whole new way of looking at my body, one that included supplements, preventive care, and the idea that small choices now protect my future.

Jessica's gift is connecting the dots. She does not see stroke, dementia, diabetes, heart disease, and hormonal issues as separate problems. She sees them as different branches of the same tree. The roots are things like inflammation, blood sugar, blood pressure, stress, and poor sleep. If you take care of the roots, you protect the branches and the tree.

That perspective gave me hope. It reminded me that I am not powerless and that the same daily habits that help me now will also protect me later.

Here are some powerful lessons that Jessica Brewer entrusted to us to share with you.

Lesson One: Start with the Gut

The very first thing Jessica asked me about was digestion. She explained that if your gut is unbalanced, nothing else in your body can function as it should. A healthy digestive system is the foundation for energy, blood sugar control, and even mental clarity.

Solution: Build meals around fiber-rich foods such as leafy greens, beans, and whole grains. Include fermented foods like yogurt, kefir, or sauerkraut. Drink plenty of water and cut back on highly processed snacks that disrupt the gut.

Lesson Two: The Roots of Disease

Jessica helped me see that stroke, dementia, diabetes, and heart disease are not separate battles. They are branches of the same tree. The roots of that tree are inflammation, high blood sugar, uncontrolled blood pressure, chronic stress, and poor sleep. If you tend to the roots, the branches stay strong.

Solution: Protect the roots with anti-inflammatory foods such as berries, leafy greens, nuts, and olive oil. Keep your blood sugar steady, monitor your blood pressure, and make room for both movement and rest.

Lesson Three: Prevention Begins Early

I used to think prevention was something you worried about later in life, but Jessica showed me that these conditions build silently for decades. High blood pressure, high blood sugar, and weight gain often start long before the first symptom appears.

Solution: Begin now, no matter your age. Know your numbers, pay attention to your choices, and view prevention as a gift to your future self.

Lesson Four: Supplements as Tools

Jessica believes modern food cannot meet all of our nutritional needs. Our soil has been stripped of minerals, and our diets are rushed and processed. Supplements can help bridge the gap. She often highlights magnesium, vitamin D, omega-3 fatty acids, probiotics, and B vitamins as essential for brain and body health. I take all of them.

She also notes that in some countries, CoQ10 is required when statins are prescribed because statins can deplete the body's natural stores of CoQ10. Without it, muscle pain, weakness, and fatigue can follow. Supplementing with CoQ10 can protect energy, heart function, and brain health.

Solution: Do not guess when it comes to supplements. Work with a professional who can guide you on what your body specifically needs. Choose quality and see supplements as helpers, not replacements for food.

Quick note: Both Jerome and Jessica remind us that how we live and what we eat have changed in ways that deeply affect our health. Our grandparents often grew food in backyard gardens or bought produce from nearby farms. Meals were made from whole ingredients, cooked slowly, and shared around a table.

Today, much of what fills our plates comes from large-scale production. Processed and packaged foods travel hundreds or even thousands of miles before reaching our kitchens. In the United States, studies show that more than 60 percent of the average diet now comes from ultra-processed foods, which are made with refined grains, added sugars, seed oils, and preservatives. These foods are engineered for shelf life and flavor, not for nourishment.

The soil that once produced nutrient-dense vegetables has also changed. Modern farming relies heavily on chemical fertilizers and monocropping, practices that deplete minerals such as magnesium and zinc. As a result, the fruits and vegetables we eat today often contain 20 to 40 percent fewer nutrients than those grown just fifty years ago.

This shift means we must be more intentional about how we eat. Choosing fresh, seasonal foods, cooking at home, and supporting local farms can help bring back the richness that once came naturally. Supplements can fill some gaps, but they cannot replace the vitality of real food grown in healthy soil.

In short, the table has changed, but our bodies have not. They still crave what the earth was meant to provide… food that is close to its source, prepared with care, and eaten with gratitude.

Lesson Five: Looking Ahead

Jessica is not afraid to explore new therapies, but she is careful and thoughtful about them. She told me about vagus nerve stimulation, a treatment already approved for migraines that may soon be approved for post-stroke recovery. She also spoke about the ketogenic diet, which may reduce brain inflammation and protect neurons, though she reminds us that more research is needed.

Solution: Stay curious, stay open, and keep asking questions. Explore new options, always with guidance and care.

Jessica Brewer's Brain Health Protocol

Jessica created this protocol for Alzheimer's prevention, yet every step also protects against stroke and strengthens recovery. What helps memory also protects circulation, mobility, and overall quality of life.

- Know your numbers: Monitor blood pressure, blood sugar, cholesterol, and kidney function. Healthy ranges protect the brain's blood vessels.
- Eat for your brain: Choose whole foods rich in fiber and low in added sugar. Build meals that fuel the brain and stabilize blood pressure and blood sugar.
- Move daily: Walk, stretch, or dance most days. Add strength training and short bursts of intensity when possible to improve circulation and balance.

- Prioritize sleep: Deep, restful sleep repairs the brain. If you snore or wake unrefreshed, screen for sleep apnea.

- Manage stress: Calmer nervous systems protect blood vessels, improve sleep, and provide steady energy for daily life and recovery.

- Care for your teeth and gums: Good dental hygiene reduces inflammation that can increase stroke risk.

- Limit alcohol and avoid smoking: Both weaken blood vessels and increase the risk of stroke and cognitive decline.

- Stay mentally active: Read, write, play music, or do puzzles. Keep learning and connecting with others to strengthen brain networks and support healing.

- Stay socially connected and purposeful: Community and purpose foster motivation, resilience, and joy that protect both the brain and the heart.

This is not about perfection or quick fixes. It is about building steady habits that serve you over time. When we care for the brain, we also care for the heart, the body, and the future we hope to live in.

wellbeingsmedical.com
Functional and metabolic medicine specialist restoring balance from root causes

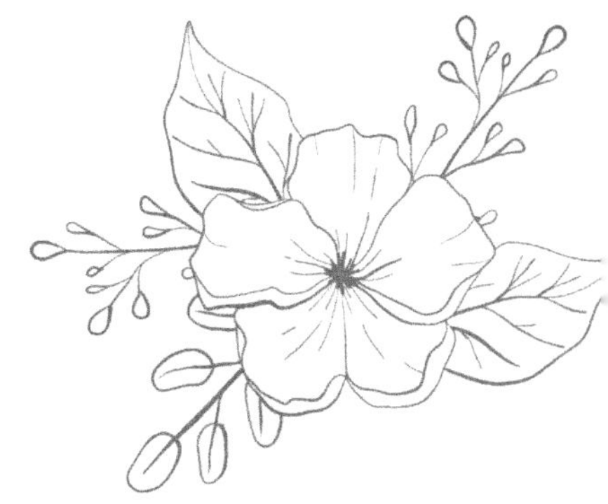

CHAPTER EIGHT

PREVENTION – BEGIN AGAIN

Taura

Eight is a number that has always carried meaning. In many faith traditions, it represents new beginnings, a fresh start, and rising after the fall. When we think about prevention, we are really talking about the blessing of starting again. Another day to make better choices, another walk around the block, another meal that fuels the body instead of fighting it. The gift of again is not guaranteed, which is why it must be treasured.

From my mother's story and my own, we have learned that prevention is not punishment. It is love in action. Each choice toward wellness is hope deposited into a wealthy life savings account. It's another chance to sing, to laugh, and to see the people you love grow into themselves. It's another chance to change the story that strokes often try to write for us.

This chapter is about those choices, the ones that help protect the mind, the heart, and the body. It is about the daily practices that may seem small but hold the power to rewrite an ending. It is about remembering that every tomorrow is a gift and that prevention is how we unwrap it.

Family History

Family history matters, but it does not tell the whole story. We often hear, "It runs in my family," as if the outcome has already been decided. The truth is more complex. Yes, genetics play a role in stroke risk, but lifestyle choices such as how we eat, move, rest, and respond to stress can influence how those inherited traits show up in our lives. Scientists call this epigenetics, the idea that our environment and daily practices can switch certain genes on or off. That means prevention is not just possible; it is powerful.

If stroke runs in your family line, you are not bound to repeat it. Prevention offers you another chance to shift the outcome, rewrite the pattern, and live beyond what your family history might suggest. Each step you take toward health is a step away from a destiny that seems fixed but is not.

Being informed also makes a difference. Knowing your numbers, risks, and options allow you to make choices from a place of power rather than fear. The more you understand your body and your family history, the better prepared you are to change the story.

When Lifestyle Choices Outperformed Family History

In a study of more than 300,000 adults in the United Kingdom, people with an unfavorable lifestyle had a 66 percent higher risk of stroke than those with healthier habits, and this was true at every level of genetic risk. Lifestyle and genes acted independently, meaning healthy choices lowered risk even for those at high genetic risk.

Another long-term study followed adults in midlife and found that those who practiced what is known as Life's Simple 7, which includes managing blood pressure, controlling cholesterol, reducing blood sugar, staying active, eating better, losing weight, and stopping smoking, had about a 30 to 43 percent lower lifetime risk of stroke across all genetic levels. In other words, better cardiovascular health partly offset a high inherited risk.

Research also shows that for people with high blood pressure, a healthy lifestyle reduces stroke risk by about 30 percent, regardless of genetic background. In fact, those with high genetic risk who lived healthfully often had a lower absolute stroke risk over twelve years than people with lower genetic risk who lived unhealthfully.

Smoking cessation is another powerful example. Former smokers quickly lower their stroke risk after quitting. Studies have found that the risk drops by roughly one-third compared with those who continue smoking, and within about five-years it can approach the risk level of people who never smoked.

Diet also makes a difference. People who followed a Mediterranean-style eating pattern, rich in fruits, vegetables, fish, whole grains, and healthy oils, were less likely to experience stroke, even when other risks were present.

Blood pressure control may be one of the most significant factors. Across many trials, each 10 mmHg (ten millimeters of mercury) drop in systolic blood pressure was associated with a 27 percent reduction in stroke risk. In one landmark study, a treatment combining blood pressure medications reduced the risk of recurrent stroke by 43 percent among those who had already experienced one. Family history did not diminish these benefits.

A gentle reminder: lifestyle does not rewrite your DNA sequence, but through epigenetics it can influence whether genes are turned on or off. This is one of the reasons healthy choices can mitigate inherited risk.

My mom will touch more on blood pressure monitoring , but I wanted to share tests and screenings that you might want to request from your doctor, which may help you assess your risk for stroke.

- **Hemoglobin A1c** – Shows average blood sugar levels over the past two to three months. Elevated levels indicate diabetes or pre-diabetes, both of which significantly increase stroke risk.
- **Fasting Blood Glucose** – Measures real-time blood sugar control and helps identify insulin resistance.

- **Lipid Panel (Cholesterol Test)** – Assesses total cholesterol, LDL, HDL, and triglycerides. High levels can lead to plaque buildup in arteries.

- **C Reactive Protein (CRP or hs CRP)** – Indicates inflammation in the body, which is linked to vascular damage and stroke risk.

- **Complete Blood Count (CBC)** – Evaluates red and white blood cells and platelets. Abnormalities can affect circulation, oxygen delivery, or clotting.

- **Coagulation Panel (PT, INR, aPTT)** – Measures how well blood clots. Overactive clotting raises stroke risk.

- **Fibrinogen** – A protein involved in clot formation. Elevated levels increase the likelihood of clots.

- **Homocysteine** – High levels are associated with increased cardiovascular and stroke risk.

- **Lipoprotein(a)** – A genetic cholesterol marker that can increase stroke risk even when standard cholesterol levels appear normal.

- **D Dimer** – Signals recent or ongoing clot activity and may prompt further imaging.

Other Important Screenings

- **Electrocardiogram (EKG or ECG)** – Detects heart rhythm irregularities such as atrial fibrillation.

- **Carotid Ultrasound** – Evaluates plaque or narrowing in arteries supplying blood to the brain.

- **CT or MRI of the Brain (when indicated)** – Identifies prior strokes, bleeding, or **structural risk factors.**

Please remember that you can take every test and preventative measure in the world and still have a stroke. Prevention lowers risk, but does not offer guarantees…such is life.

KNOW PRESSURE

Yvonne

Taura just mentioned that blood pressure control is one of the most significant risk factors, and I could not agree more. As I mentioned before, I was unaware that I had high blood pressure, but I check it often now and use blood pressure medication to stay on top of it. Prevention still matters to me, even as a survivor, because I do not want another stroke.

Here are some of the things that can raise blood pressure, and some of the things that help bring it down:

What makes blood pressure rise

- Too much salt in our food
- Too much sugar
- Processed meals that are quick but not nutritious
- Weight gain and lack of regular movement
- Stress and carrying too many worries
- Lack of rest or poor sleep
- Medical conditions such as diabetes or kidney disease
- Family history of high blood pressure

What helps lower blood pressure

- Checking it often and keeping track of the numbers.
- Taking prescribed medication regularly
- Eating more fresh foods and cutting back on salt and sugar
- Moving the body every day, even if it is just walking
- Finding ways to ease stress, such as prayer, breathing, or music
- Getting good rest and giving the body time to recover
- Staying on top of other health conditions with regular checkups

(Reading for my mom)

I also believe people have to do what works for them. For me, that means I am not ashamed to take life-saving medication, but I also like to pair it with simple remedies I can use at home. One thing I do every morning is take apple cider vinegar. It helps with digestion, feeds the good bacteria in the gut, and keeps my stomach and energy more balanced. I also keep baking soda close by. A small amount in water can calm stomach acid and help me feel steady. These might seem like little things, but they are part of what works for me.

It is also important to know what high blood pressure feels like. For me, it has shown up in ways I did not expect. You may experience headaches that will not go away, dizziness or blurred vision, shortness of breath, chest pain or a pounding feeling in the chest, neck, or ears. Some people notice nosebleeds or feel unusually tired and confused. The tricky thing is that high blood pressure does not always show symptoms, which is why checking it often is so important.

I know prevention is not the same for everyone, but I believe in using every tool available. For me, that means taking my medicine, checking my blood pressure, and trusting a few natural remedies that give me comfort and strength. I did not know how important this was until it was almost too late. Now I know that controlling blood pressure is one of the strongest tools we have to prevent strokes from occurring in the first place or from recurring.

PRESSURE CHECK

I have learned that it is not enough to hope my blood pressure is under control; I have to check it. I keep an upper-arm cuff at home, which most doctors recommend because it is the most accurate. And I write my numbers down so I can notice changes over time.

Here are some devices that may help you to monitor your blood pressure more effectively.

- **Upper-arm cuff monitors** remain the gold standard at home. They are easy to use and provide reliable readings.

- **Wrist monitors** can work too, especially for people who find arm cuffs uncomfortable, but you have to use them carefully to get good results.

- **Smartwatches** like the Apple Watch and Samsung Galaxy Watch do not replace a cuff, but they can alert you to heart rate changes and keep you aware of your health throughout the day.

- **Smart rings** – some track blood pressure, but they are still new and not always accurate. They may be useful for tracking trends, but not for medical decisions.

- **Specialized devices** like the Omron HeartGuide, which looks like a watch, and the Withings BPM Core, which connects to your phone, combine convenience with medical accuracy.

For me, I keep my cuff at home and sometimes I use my watch to keep an eye on my heart rate. What matters most is finding something you will actually use. Prevention works when we stay aware and consistent. I also want you to know that you do not have to spend a lot of money to keep track of your numbers. Many drugstores and pharmacies offer free blood pressure monitors that anyone can use. If you are out running errands, you can take a few minutes to sit down and check your pressure. It is a simple way to stay aware, and for some people, it is the only chance they get to see their numbers.

Checks and Balances

Taura

This chapter is about awareness. We don't want to overwhelm you with too much repetition, but we also don't want you to miss that there are many ways to check in on your health. Not every test is right for everyone, but knowing what's out there can help you feel more informed when you sit across from a doctor.

If we sound repetitive, sorry, not sorry. We want and need you to "get it"! We're sharing these options so you know what's available. Everybody is different, and not every test, process or screening is right for you per sé, so please always talk with your doctor and find your perfect fit.

A Personal Note

After recovering from Covid, my heart began racing in a way I had never experienced before. It alarmed me so much that I went to the Tarzana Cardiac Center, where the doctors ran a series of tests: a stress test, an echocardiogram, an ECG, and a carotid ultrasound. Every result came back normal. They told me it was likely anxiety mixed with my body's unknown reaction to the virus.

The doctors also suggested that I consider a heart-healthy vegetarian diet, which I am just beginning to explore. I felt empowered walking away…not only with reassurance but also with new tools for prevention.

That experience taught me how easily anxiety can mimic the symptoms of a heart attack or even a stroke, such as a racing heart, shortness of breath, dizziness, or chest tightness. The key difference is, anxiety symptoms often come in waves and may ease with calming, deep breathing or grounding. Stroke and heart attack symptoms, on the other hand, usually do not let up and often come with sudden, severe changes: numbness, weakness, slurred speech, drooping face, or crushing chest pain.

Still, the only safe choice is to **get checked**. Let the doctors decide. If you notice something different in your body and it scares you, do not second-guess yourself. Anxiety can be managed, but a stroke or heart attack requires immediate attention.

Quick Comparison: Anxiety vs. Stroke/Heart Attack

Anxiety	Stroke / Heart Attack
Symptoms may come and go in waves	Symptoms are sudden, severe, and persistent
Often linked to stress, fear, or panic	Can occur without warning, even at rest
May improve with calming, breathing, or grounding	Do not improve with calming techniques

Anxiety	Stroke / Heart Attack
Fast heartbeat, dizziness, sweating, chest tightness	Facial drooping, slurred speech, weakness, and/or crushing chest pain

Gratitude > Stress

Yvonne

Stress is not just an emotion. Research shows it is one of the most powerful stroke triggers. Studies have found that people who live with chronic stress are at higher risk of high blood pressure, heart disease, and stroke. The American Heart Association notes that stress hormones like cortisol can damage blood vessels over time, and that unrelieved tension can silently raise risk. This is real, and it affects us more than we sometimes want to admit.

I will admit that I am guilty of keeping things in. I hold on to hurt, carry my worries, and pretend to be strong when I might need support or to express my feelings. That is not healthy. It is hard not to feel stressed when you do not have a place to lay your head or when you do not know where your next meal will come from. Life has not always been easy, and life after a stroke isn't easy. It's important to note that some changes that occur after a stroke are not necessarily your fault. More on that later.

But if you are reading this book, you have hands to hold it and eyes that work. If you are listening to this book, you have ears to hear it. If you are experiencing this book through Braille or American Sign Language, you still have the gift of understanding it in a way that reaches you. And if someone is reading it to you, you have ears to hear and hope to anchor to. That means there is still something to be grateful for. Grateful that we woke up this morning. Grateful for the present moment, and every waking moment to come.

And I am so grateful that I stand firm on Jeremiah 29:11, and have found peace and joy in the waiting.

BREATHE

Now let's take another breath break. Breathe in slowly, as if you are filling a balloon deep in your belly. Hold it for a moment, then let it out gently, as if you are blowing through a straw.

Do it again, noticing how your body softens with each release. This simple act is a reminder that even when life feels heavy, we can choose to pause, breathe, and release some of the pressure.

Taura

Woosah!

When my mom was recovering, it was so hard to find information that spoke to me. I spent so much time googling, and you know how that goes. Rabbit holes don't always lead to the best information. Everything was so bleak and scary, which brings us to this very moment. Writing this book together, which I am extremely grateful for.

Let It Out

I want to talk about what it means to let it out. My mom and I attended therapy sessions during her recovery, and it was not easy. Sharing a home with someone can be a challenge, even when that someone is your own mother or daughter. Add to that the changes in your body and mind after a stroke, and it can feel overwhelming. We went through a hard season, one I sometimes wish I could erase. But the blessing is that maybe you are going through something similar, and now you know you are not alone.

My mom and I communicated in very different ways. Learning to speak someone else's language, or at least understand how they express themselves, changes everything. That lesson holds true even when you are not living under the same roof.

Letting it out does not always mean sitting in a formal office. Sometimes, the friends who truly listen and respond with care offer a form of therapy, too. When words heal, encourage, and help you move forward, that is therapy in its own way.

There are many ways to find support now. It might be by phone, through telehealth, on Zoom, or in person. However it happens, it is always a good idea to talk to someone. Not everyone can afford regular sessions, but therapy is covered by most insurance plans, including Medicare. If Medicare covers it, that should tell you how important it is. For those without insurance, there are still community programs and organizations that can help. You do not have to carry it all alone.

Because therapy is part of recovery, it helps not only with stress, anxiety, and depression but also with the physical healing process after a stroke. Taking care of your mind supports your body as well. The following resources are a place to begin:

- **American Stroke Association** – Offers stroke-specific resources, education, and support groups for survivors and caregivers.

- **Family Caregiver Alliance** – A trusted guide for caregivers navigating stroke recovery transitions from hospital to home, with strategies and referrals.

- **The Loveland Foundation Therapy Fund** – Financial assistance for Black women and nonbinary individuals seeking culturally competent therapy (4 to 12 sessions).

- **Therapy for Black Girls** – An online community and directory focused on the mental wellness of Black women and girls, with both therapist listings and supportive content.

- **Free Black Therapy** – A nonprofit connecting individuals with free virtual sessions from Black therapists.

- **Women's Emotional Wellness Center** – Comprehensive services including individual therapy, group programs, and psychiatric care for women of all backgrounds.

- **Grief Counseling Resources** – Available through many hospitals, hospices, and community centers. Organizations like GriefShare and local faith communities offer group and individual counseling for those coping with loss.

- **NAMI (National Alliance on Mental Illness)** – Provides peer support, education programs, and resources for individuals and caregivers nationwide.

- **BEAM (Black Emotional and Mental Health Collective)** – Offers training, culturally responsive resources, and community-based emotional wellness for Black individuals.

POST STROKE PERSONAILITY CHANGES

It is important to be gentle with a loved one who has had a stroke because they may not necessarily have control over many of the changes they are facing. According to the American Stroke Association, a stroke can affect the parts of the brain responsible for emotion regulation, impulse control, and communication. What may appear as anger is often rooted in frustration, confusion, or the exhaustion of trying to process and express thoughts. Withdrawal and periods of silence are common because conversation can require significantly more mental effort after a stroke. Emotional spiraling, where feelings intensify quickly and feel unmanageable, can occur when the brain struggles to regulate emotional responses the way it once did. Anxiety, tearfulness, irritability, and sudden mood shifts are well-documented effects of stroke-related brain injury and are not intentional behavior.

I did not know this at the time, and I was often frustrated with my mom for going completely silent or lashing out and then seeming to forget about it altogether. It was a tough time, and I thought her reactions were about me. Now I see more clearly that she was the one having the hardest time. Most of us cannot simply reboot our computers, so imagine how challenging it must be to restart, refresh, or reconfigure the brain itself. As caregivers, patience matters. Try not to take these changes personally. At the same time, there is a responsibility to gently guide your loved one away from behaviors that are harmful to them or to the people who love them, always leading with compassion and understanding.

Here a few tips…

Handling Post Stroke Changes with Care

Anger or irritability
Anger after a stroke often stems from frustration, confusion, or fatigue. Stay calm and avoid arguing in the moment. Give space

when needed and return to the conversation later, when emotions have settled.

Withdrawal or silence

Conversation can require much more mental effort after a stroke. Allow quiet without pressure while continuing to offer gentle connection through presence, simple questions, or shared activities.

Emotional spiraling

Feelings may rise quickly and feel unmanageable because the brain struggles to regulate emotional responses. Acknowledge the feelings without trying to fix them right away. Slow the moment down and reduce noise or stimulation.

Mood swings

Sudden shifts from calm to sadness or anger are common. Do not take these changes personally. Consistent routines and a calm environment can help reduce emotional overload.

Anxiety or fearfulness

Many stroke survivors experience heightened anxiety about health, safety, or independence. Offer reassurance, explain things clearly, and maintain predictable routines. Encourage professional support if anxiety interferes with daily life.

Depression or prolonged sadness

Depression is common after stroke and may be neurological, emotional, or both. Watch for prolonged sadness, withdrawal, or loss of interest, and seek medical or mental health support early.

Impulsivity or reduced emotional filter

The ability to pause before reacting may be affected. Set gentle boundaries, redirect when needed, and prioritize safety without shame or punishment.

Fatigue and overwhelm

Mental and emotional fatigue can appear suddenly. Build in rest, shorten conversations, and allow breaks without guilt. Healing requires energy and patience.

Lose Wait (W-A-I-T)

Taura

I borrowed this sub-topic from my first book, *100 THINGS EV-ERY BLACK GIRL SHOULD KNOW: FOR GIRLS 10–100*. It was a chapter title in that book and almost the title of this book, but we landed on *THE GIFT OF AGAIN* because what a beautiful gift it is to say I love you again, to start again, to try again… It's a powerful message we hope will resonate with every reader. But the title *LOSE WAIT* is more directive, less gentle, yet still extremely important, because procrastination is probably the most crowded nation of them all.

To be completely transparent, it's 12:56 p.m., and I scheduled myself to be at the gym at noon. A couple of calls came in that derailed my plans, and now I won't go until later this afternoon. That's progress, because there have been many seasons when I wouldn't go at all. The older you get, like me, the more you see that not going is no longer an option, and that's just from a health perspective. But procrastination creeps into every crevice of our lives, and before you know it, it's all gone. The business opportunity, the ability, the guy, or the girl.

I wrote in *100 THINGS EVERY BLACK GIRL SHOULD KNOW*:
"Procrastination kills more goals and dreams than failure ever will."

And to be brutally honest, I needed to hear that again. There have been so many missed opportunities, not because of them but because of me. I've finally started to take my health and weight more seriously, but along the way, there were people who wanted to help me, and I wasn't fully showing up. I'm sharing that with you in hopes that you do not make the same mistake. The weight of waiting weighs a ton and you are essentially working against yourself. When you put off the doctor's appointment, when you put off going to the gym, when you feel the lump and convince yourself that it's nothing, when you feel kind of off but wait until you can barely stand to go to the doctor or therapist.

Work can be one of the heaviest places where procrastination shows up. Stress and work are dance partners, and too many of us stay at the party long after the music has stopped. I just talked to a friend who hates her job and wants to quit. LOSE WAIT. Another friend has an incredible business idea but has not written it down. LOSE WAIT. Someone else feels silenced in meetings and keeps avoiding asking for the promotion she deserves. LOSE WAIT. Free yourself from the weight of wait and just do it. Do it now.

Yesterday, I had to have a difficult conversation and decide to remove myself from something that people I love were passionate about, but for me, it brought nothing but stress and anxiety. Because of that, I carried a stress headache for days. But the moment I finally expressed my feelings and exited peacefully, my body began to normalize. That is the power of releasing what weighs you down.

Stress is not just an emotional thief; it is a physical one. The toll it takes on your body is real, and it shows up in ways we often ignore until it is too late. Studies confirm that chronic stress can lead to high blood pressure, heart disease, and even strokes. In fact, work-related stress is now recognized as one of the leading contributors to poor health outcomes worldwide. Nearly one in three strokes is linked to preventable factors such as unmanaged stress, high blood pressure, and lifestyle habits. We cannot afford to keep waiting, hoping things will change on their own.

LOSE WAIT

Losing the wait is about refusing to stay stuck in cycles that harm you. Whether it is a job that steals your joy, a work environment that breaks your spirit, or a dream you keep putting off, every day you wait is another weight on your shoulders. And you deserve to be light enough to move, to breathe, to live fully.

Procrastination is the enemy of progress. You will be tired, but you have to move. That applies to stroke survivors and caregivers. It also applies to prevention, because the Bible reminds us in Proverbs 13:4 (ESV): *THE SOUL OF THE SLUGGARD CRAVES AND GETS NOTHING, WHILE THE SOUL OF THE DILIGENT*

IS RICHLY SUPPLIED. Please do not mistake this for us saying you should not rest. Rest is vital. But we are called to pursue what inspires us, heals us, grows us, and strengthens us with tenacity. Lose wait… what are you waiting for?

Truth moment. We have wanted to release this book for a while, but I did not feel I had lost enough weight to speak publicly about health and wellness. I have carried extra weight most of my life, and while I have made incredible progress, there is still a journey ahead. GLP-1 medications helped, but they were not permission slips to eat whatever I wanted. These medicines work with the body by mimicking a natural gut hormone that slows how quickly the stomach empties, so you feel full longer. They also calm hunger signals in the brain and help balance blood sugar by increasing insulin and lowering glucagon. In short, they gave me a real fighting chance, but I still had responsibility. I became more intentional than ever about tracking macros, knowing what nourishes my body, and choosing foods with purpose. Many of the recipes in the back of this book were born from that same intentionality, shaped by both my mother's stroke recovery and my own weight journey.

Still, I compared myself to Instagram models or to the endless stream of beautifully fit women in Los Angeles, and I felt inadequate. I wondered how people would receive this prevention and healing message when my body does not reflect medical ideals. So I paused. I healed. I unlearned the harmful stories ingrained in me.

When Oprah and doctors named obesity a disease, it felt like liberation. I had tried everything, and this treatment finally helped me send the right messages to my body. If you are reading this, do what you must to speak the same language as your body and your spirit. Then you will normalize, heal, and thrive, no matter how others see it.

I still have goals of losing more weight, building muscle, and strengthening my emotions and my connection to God. But that does not mean I have to wait to share how far I have come. My mother has walked a powerful healing path, and to me she is the living image of full recovery. Someone somewhere may not resonate with her story or mine, and that is okay. What matters is that we share our truths and encourage you find and live in your own.

Closing Reflection

Yvonne

Leaving it on the altar is not our only resource. God wants us to help one another on our journeys. Prayer is powerful, but so is fellowship. We are not meant to carry our burdens alone, and part of God's plan is that we walk alongside one another. Talking to pastors or church council can be a safe place, too.

I know that *CHURCH HURT* is real, and I have had my share of it. If you do not feel you can talk to your pastors or do not have someone safe to advise and counsel you in your church, it may be time to look for another spiritual home.

Taura

Sometimes God sends us help through other people, and sometimes those people are therapists. We have to be open enough to receive it. I know not everyone is comfortable with traditional therapy, and that is perfectly fine. Whether it is a trusted friend, a pastor, or a counselor, what matters most is that the voice you lean on is rooted in love and can offer thoughtful, unbiased guidance. If you want my recipe for healing and undoing, it is a bit of my mom's grace and watching her relentlessly serve, blended with Sarah Jakes Roberts, an endless stream of positive quotes from my sister and besties, heavy Mel Robbins podcast binges, reading or listening to Joe Dispenza, Pastor Andrea Humphrey's Hump Free Wednesdays, spending time with people who water me, and just a little bit of angsty or inspiring 90's hip hop to balance it all.

There comes a point when you have to call procrastination what it is…a terrible partner! If you wait for what is meant for now, it may not be there later. You cannot rise when you are carrying the weight of delay and doubt. *Lose the wait* so you can lift off and rise up.

The Spirit of Love

Yvonne

Before we put on aprons and head into the recipe section, we want to thank you all for reading *THE GIFT OF AGAIN*. We hope it will be a bedside and pocketbook companion for stroke survivors and caregivers for generations. Every time someone opens this book or listens to our voices, it becomes a gift to them and to us.

We also wanted to speak to how the Spirit has guided this text. Emiko had a doctor who did not fit the description of anyone on staff. Tymiak had an encounter with God. Mindy's sister-in-law felt an urgency to answer her phone. And unshakable faith guided Tracey, Clarence, and me toward healing.

Taura

What we have come to understand is this. Spirit does not speak in one language. It meets us where we are. It speaks through instinct, timing, warning, peace, and clarity. It speaks through the body when something feels off and through the heart when something feels right. These are not accidents. They are invitations to listen more closely.

If there were one scripture that encapsulates the spirit of this text, it would be Matthew 22:39, *LOVE YOUR NEIGHBOR AS YOUR-SELF*. Your gay neighbor. Your straight neighbor. Your Christian, Catholic, Baptist, Jewish, Muslim, Hindu, or agnostic neighbor. Because often times someone's world may be completely dark until they see the light in you.

Yvonne

We believe love is the common thread, and we hope to find our way back to it. Not by removing the omnipresence of God, but by remembering it. If God is love and God is everywhere, then God is in me and in you.

Taura

As 1 John 4:16 says, "And so we know and rely on the love God has for us. God is love. Whoever lives in love lives in God, and God in them."

That truth invites us to listen more closely to the voice of love within us, the quiet guidance that nudges us toward compassion, patience, self-care, and care for others. When we honor that voice, it shows up not only in what we believe but also in how we move through the world, in the way we speak to one another, in the grace we offer, and in the choices we make when no one is watching. Love becomes visible through action, and that is where healing begins.

Yvonne

That love calls us to treat one another with respect, care, and dignity.

At some point, we will all need grace. We will all need help. We will all need to borrow a cup of sugar. And perhaps the greatest gift of again is opening our eyes. To see another day, and to see with the eyes of love. To recognize spirit at work around us and within us, and to answer it with care.

CHAPTER NINE

PLATE PREP

Before we get into the recipes, we want to make sure you know how to shop for them. When you are out at a restaurant, you should feel just as prepared. Learning how to read a label, choose the right ingredients, and understand what goes into your meals gives you the recipe for success every single day. These tools make eating at home easier and help you stay on track when life takes you outside your kitchen.

This section will walk you through the basics: how to read carbs and sugars on a label, how sweeteners and fruit spreads work in your body, how to shop with confidence, and how to order with intention when you eat out. Once you understand these simple foundations, every recipe becomes easier, every choice becomes clearer, and you gain the freedom to enjoy food without guessing.

Shopping for the Life You Want

Before you start cooking, you need to know how to shop. The grocery store can either support your goals or work against them. Packaging is designed to sell you, and labels are designed to inform you. Once you understand the difference, everything becomes easier. Some of this may be a recap, and that is intentional, because the ultimate test is changing the way you eat every day. There will be plenty of pop-up quizzes along the way, and they come in the form of the choices you make at home, in the store, and out in the world. Repetition builds success.

Macros

Every food you buy contains protein, carbohydrates, and fat. These are your macros. Understanding them helps you build meals that support your energy and your hunger throughout the day. Protein supports strength and recovery. Healthy fats support hormones and satisfaction. Carbohydrates provide energy, but quality matters. Whole-food carbs work with your body. Sugary and starchy carbs often work against it.

Hidden Sugars

Sugar hides under many names. Cane sugar, brown rice syrup, fruit concentrate, agave, coconut sugar, maple syrup, maltose, and many others show up in foods that seem harmless. Even organic products can contain large amounts of sugar. If sugar is one of the first three ingredients, leave it on the shelf. If a food is high in added sugar and low in fiber, it will hit your bloodstream quickly and leave you craving more.

Honey is natural and full of flavor, but it raises your glycemic index and can cause a sharper spike in blood sugar. Agave has a lower glycemic index than honey, but it is still a form of sugar and should be used sparingly. Maple syrup is also natural but very concentrated, so a little goes a long way. Monk fruit sweetener is usually the gentlest option because it does not raise blood sugar and adds sweetness without calories. Maple syrup, agave, and date syrup are often seen as more natural alternatives to white sugar, but they are still high in sugar and should be used in moderation. Maple syrup is concentrated and high in natural sugars, which means it can raise blood glucose levels quickly if used in larger amounts. Agave has a lower glycemic index than many sweeteners, but it is high in fructose and can still impact blood sugar and metabolic health when overused. Date syrup is made from whole dates and contains small amounts of fiber and nutrients, but it can also cause blood sugar spikes, especially for those managing glucose. These sweeteners can add flavor and depth, but portion size matters. If you are watching your glucose, monk fruit is the safest and most consistent choice in the group. This doesn't mean you can't eat any of these ever again; moderation and space are key. Syrup over the weekend with whole-wheat or gluten-free pancakes? Sure, but even if you top lettuce with syrup, sugar, or honey every day, your body probably wouldn't like it very much.

Jams and jellies follow the same rules. Organic does not automatically mean healthy. Many fruit spreads, even organic ones, are still high in sugar or made from concentrates. If a product is heavily processed, your body has to work harder to break it down. Look for spreads made from whole fruit, with no added sugar and the fewest ingredients possible. Small choices like these support you every day.

ORGANIC

Organic means the ingredients were grown without certain chemicals. It does not mean the food is good for your heart or your recovery. Organic cookies are still cookies. Organic jelly is still sugar. Do not let the word organic make choices for you. The ingredient list always tells the truth.

Do Not Drink Your Calories

Drinks are one of the most common places where hidden sugar hides. Smoothies, juices, flavored coffees, sweet teas, and bottled "health" drinks often contain more sugar than dessert. Your body does not process liquid calories the same way it processes food, so you take in more without feeling full. Choose water, herbal tea, or flavored water with no added sugar most of the time.

Ingredients Matter

Short ingredient lists are almost always better. A long list with unfamiliar terms is a sign of heavy processing. Your body has to work harder to break down these additives, and many can trigger inflammation. Look for ingredients you recognize and could use at home.

Oils to Avoid

Many packaged foods contain oils that work against your health goals. These include soybean oil, corn oil, canola oil, cottonseed oil, vegetable oil, and palm oil. They appear in dressings, crackers, frozen meals, sauces, and even foods that appear healthy.

Hydrogenated and partially hydrogenated oils are even more important to avoid. These oils are chemically altered to stay solid and shelf-stable, making them very difficult for your body to break down. They can affect your heart, circulation, and inflammation levels.

Choose items made with olive oil or avocado oil when possible, or foods that do not require added oils at all.

Watch the Sodium

Salt is hidden in many foods that do not taste salty. Frozen meals, canned soups, breads, sauces, dressings, and almost all restaurant food can contain very high amounts of sodium. Too much sodium affects your heart, your blood pressure, and your overall recovery. Compare brands and choose lower-sodium versions when you can. Small changes make a big difference over time.

Understanding the Nutrition Label

Most people glance at a nutrition label without really knowing what they are looking at. When you understand each part, you can make choices that support your daily life instead of guessing. Here is how to read the sections that matter most.

Serving

This is the first number to look at. If the serving size is ½ cup and you eat a full cup, you must double every number on the label. Many people eat two or three servings without realizing it, which changes everything.

Carbohydrates

Carbs include starches, sugars, fiber, and sugar alcohols. What matters most is how many carbs your body treats as sugar. To calculate net carbs, start with Total Carbohydrates, subtract Dietary Fiber, then subtract approved sugar alcohols such as erythritol. Do not subtract sugar alcohols that raise blood sugar, including maltitol, isomalt, and maltodextrin.

Example:
Total carbs: 22
Fiber: 5
Sugar alcohol (erythritol): 6
22 − 5 − 6 = 11 net carbs

Sugars

Under carbohydrates, you will see Total Sugars and Added Sugars. Total Sugars includes what is naturally present in fruit and dairy. Added Sugars is the most important number because it is the sugar the company added to the product. If added sugar is high and fiber is low, the food will hit your bloodstream quickly.

Fiber

Fiber helps with fullness, digestion, and blood sugar control. More fiber is usually better. It also lowers your net carbs, which is why it is an important number to track.

Fats

Not all fats are the same. Saturated fat should be consumed in moderation. Trans fat should be avoided completely. If a label says 0 grams of trans fat but the ingredients list hydrogenated or partially hydrogenated oil, put it back. Better fats include olive oil, avocado oil, nuts, and seeds. Oils to limit include soybean, corn, cottonseed, vegetable, and palm oil.

Protein

Protein supports recovery, strength, and blood sugar stability. If a meal or snack is too low in protein, you will feel hungry again soon after. Look for foods with a significant amount of protein, not just one or two grams.

Sodium

Sodium is hidden in many foods that do not taste salty. High sodium levels affect blood pressure and overall heart health. When comparing similar items, choose the one with lower sodium.

Cholesterol

For many people, dietary cholesterol is less of a concern than saturated fat and sodium, but always follow your doctor's guidance if you have heart or circulation concerns.

Ingredients List

This section tells the truth. Ingredients are listed in order of quantity, so if sugar is near the top, it is not a good choice. The fewer ingredients, the better. If the list is long, confusing, or filled with artificial additives, the product is heavily processed and harder for your body to handle. If you cannot pronounce an ingredient, your body will not process it easily.

Doctor's Orders

Before you make major changes to your diet, make sure your grocery list and nutrition plan align with your doctor's recommendations. Everyone's health needs are different. If you do not already have a nutrition plan from your doctor or medical professional, this is the perfect time to ask for one. Clear guidance helps you make choices that support your specific needs.

Label Do's and Don'ts Recap

Do:

- Check the serving size first
- Look at total carbs and subtract fiber
- Subtract only sugar alcohols that do not raise blood sugar, such as erythritol
- Choose foods with higher fiber and meaningful protein
- Compare sodium levels and choose the lower option
- Read the ingredient list from top to bottom
- Choose products with short, simple ingredients
- Look for whole foods instead of processed fillers
- Make sure the food fits your doctor's nutrition plan

Don't:

- Don't trust the front of the package
- Don't ignore serving size or portion math
- Don't subtract maltitol, isomalt, or maltodextrin from your carbs
- Don't buy foods where sugar or oil is among the first three ingredients
- Don't overlook hidden sugars with names like syrup, concentrate, or nectar
- Don't choose items made with hydrogenated or partially hydrogenated oils
- Don't rely on "organic" or "all natural" as a sign of health
- Don't assume a food is healthy just because it looks healthy

Dining Out with Intention

I have never been big on eating out. I have always preferred cooking at home, where I know exactly what I am making and how it makes me feel. But Taura's lifestyle puts her in restaurants all the time, and life does not slow down just because you are trying to make healthier choices. So even though I am not a restaurant person, I do have a few simple rules that can help you stay steady when you are away from your own kitchen.

Start with Protein

Most restaurants can add protein, even if it is not listed on the menu. Ask for chicken, fish, shrimp, beans, or another lean option to be added to your salad or main dish. You can also ask for egg whites instead of whole eggs at breakfast. Protein helps you stay satisfied so you do not overeat.

Potatoes Are Not the Enemy

A baked or roasted potato can be a good choice. It gives you steady energy and keeps you full. The trouble is not the potato; it is the toppings. Keep it simple. Add vegetables like spinach, broccoli, mushrooms, or peppers to make it more filling. Ask for it roasted or baked, never fried.

Watch for Hidden Fried Foods

Some dishes look healthy but are fried without being labeled as such. Brussels sprouts, cauliflower, chicken, and even some meats are often deep-fried before sauces or glazes are added. If you are unsure, ask how the dish is prepared. Choose grilled, roasted, steamed, or sautéed options instead.

Keep Rice or Pasta on the Side

Restaurants serve very large portions of rice and pasta. Ask for it on the side and add only half to your meal. This keeps your plate balanced without making you feel like you missed out.

Cut the Plate in Half

When your meal arrives, divide it in half right away and plan to take the rest home. This helps you stop when you are full, not when the plate is empty.

Dressings, Sauces, and Syrups on the Side

Ask for all dressings and sauces on the side so you control how much you use. If you order waffles, pancakes, oatmeal, or anything that usually comes with sugary syrup, ask for fresh berries instead. If you want a little sweetness, bring or request a natural sweetener you trust and add a small amount yourself.

Eat a Little Something Before You Go

Have a small protein snack at home before you leave. A boiled egg, some yogurt, or a handful of nuts helps you arrive without feeling starved, making it much easier to order mindfully.

Choose Simple Desserts

If dessert is part of the evening, opt for something light. Fresh berries with cream, a small scoop of ice cream with coffee, or sharing something with the table lets you enjoy the moment without overdoing it.

Choose Clean Cocktails

If you are having a drink, choose something simple. Clean options include red wine, vodka, or mezcal. Avoid sugary cocktails with syrups or juice. Pair each drink with a glass of water to stay balanced.

Choose Water or Unsweetened Iced Tea First

Start with water. If you want tea, choose it unsweetened and add lemon or your own sweetener if needed. Sweet teas and flavored drinks can contain more sugar than dessert.

Take Your Time

Restaurants move quickly, but you do not have to. Slow down. Enjoy the company. Put your fork down between bites. When you eat slowly, your body has time to tell you when it has had enough.

Even though I prefer my own kitchen, I know life happens outside it. With a few thoughtful habits, your restaurant meals can fit right into the way you want to live and feel.

CHAPTER TEN

THE GIFT TABLE

Taura

Now, this is where the fun begins. Recipes are personal. They tell stories, carry memories, and bring us back to the table together. There is no one size fits all menu, just like gifts. So here at the gift table, there is something for everyone. If you don't like certain ingredients, just flip the page until something calls your name!

My mom and I don't always eat the same way, but we have learned to share the kitchen and balance each other out.
I need rules when it comes to food, or I get carried away. I always say I gain weight just by standing too close to biscuits. That's why I started remixing comfort foods. I want the taste of home, but healthier.

Yvonne

I love salads. I could eat them every day, but I know a salad can go from healthy to heavy depending on the dressing. Lately, I have been having fun experimenting with new dressing recipes, using lighter oils, citrus, yogurt, and spices that add flavor without piling on calories or fat. It is a way to keep my salads exciting and good for me at the same time. Well, enough about us. Now it's time for you to try your new lifestyle out in the kitchen!

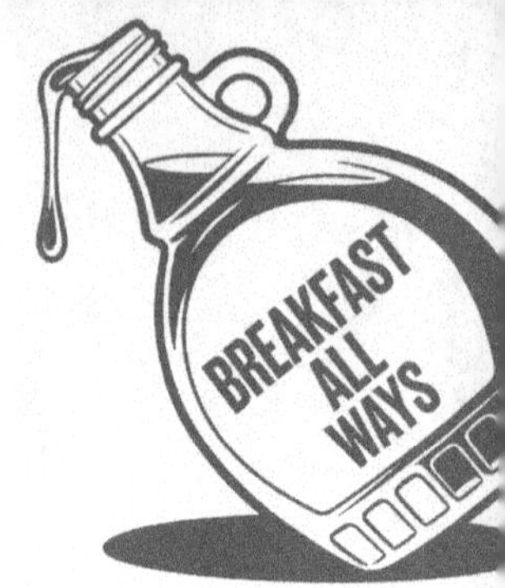

Breakfast All Ways

Von: Before my stroke, I routinely skipped breakfast, but I learned that breakfast works best for my body, even if it's just a smoothie.

Taura: Please note that breakfast does not come with a clock attached. Eat it whenever you want, to break intermittent fasting or at 3pm after lunch.

Protein Pudding with Berries

Serves 1

Ingredients

- ½ cup Greek yogurt or unsweetened plant-based yogurt
- 2 tbsp chia seeds
- 1 scoop protein powder (plain or vanilla)
- ½ cup soy milk or almond milk
- 1 tsp honey or monk fruit sweetener (optional)
- Fresh berries for topping

Directions

1. Mix yogurt, chia seeds, protein powder, and milk in a bowl or jar.

2. Stir well, cover, and refrigerate for at least 2 hours or overnight.

3. Top with fresh berries before serving.

Loaded Oatmeal

Serves 1

Ingredients

- ½ cup rolled oats
- 1 cup soy milk or almond milk
- 1 tbsp flax seeds or chia seeds
- ¼ cup almonds or walnuts
- 1 tbsp almond butter or peanut butter
- ½ banana, sliced or sliced dates, raisins or fresh blueberries
- Cinnamon to taste

Directions

1. Cook oats in milk on the stove until creamy.

2. Stir in flax seeds, nuts, and almond butter.

3. Top with banana slices and a sprinkle of cinnamon.

Grits with Kale, Mushrooms, and an Egg

Serves 2

Ingredients

- ½ cup stone-ground grits
- 2 cups water or low-sodium vegetable broth
- 1 cup kale, chopped
- ½ cup mushrooms, sliced
- 1 egg, poached or soft-fried (per serving)
- 1 tsp olive oil
- Salt and pepper to taste

Directions

1. Cook grits in water or broth until creamy.

2. In a skillet, sauté the kale and mushrooms in olive oil until tender.

3. Serve the grits topped with the greens and finish with the egg.

How Low Can You Go Smoothie?

LDL reducing smoothie!

Ingredients

- 1 apple, chopped
- ½ cup oats
- 1 cup soy protein milk
- 1 tbsp flax seeds
- ¼ cup almonds
- ⅓ cup Greek yogurt
- ½ cup berries (optional)
- A scoop of protein powder

Directions

1. Blend all ingredients until smooth.

2. Adjust thickness with more soy milk or water if needed.

3. Serve cold.

Tip: If you do not have soy protein milk or prefer to skip soy, you can use any high-protein plant milk you like. Pea, oat, or flax milk all work beautifully as long as they are unsweetened and contain about eight to ten grams of protein per cup. Brands like Ripple, Chobani Oat Extra Protein, and Good Karma are easy to find and make this recipe just as heart-healthy.

For added cholesterol-lowering power, you can blend in a small scoop of plant sterol powder, such as CholestOff, or add half a cup of cooked and drained white or black beans (and cacao) for a chocolate shake. Both options increase fiber and help support healthy cholesterol levels without changing the flavor.

SoCal Avocado Toast

Serves 1

Ingredients

- 1 ripe avocado
- ½ tsp ground cumin
- Juice of ½ lemon
- Pinch of salt + coarse salt for topping
- 2 slices whole-grain bread, toasted
- 2–3 thin slices red onion
- 2–3 thin slices red jalapeño
- 2 tbsp plant-based feta cheese
- 1 tbsp pepita seeds

Directions

1. In a small bowl, mash the avocado with cumin, lemon juice, and a pinch of salt until smooth but slightly chunky.

2. Spread mixture evenly over toasted bread.

3. Top with red onion, jalapeño slices, plant-based feta, and pepita seeds.

4. Finish with a sprinkle of coarse salt, then serve right away.

Quiana's Breakfast Burrito

Serves 1

Ingredients

- 1 flour tortilla (regular or low-carb version)
- ½ cup black beans, warmed
- ¼ avocado, sliced or mashed
- ½ cup roasted potatoes, crispy
- 2 eggs, scrambled and fluffy (or plant-based alternative)
- 2 tbsp salsa
- 2 tbsp shredded cheese (plant-based cheddar or regular, if you choose to splurge)

Directions

1. Warm the tortilla in a skillet or over an open flame until soft and pliable.

2. Layer black beans, avocado, roasted potatoes, scrambled eggs, salsa, and cheese in the center.

3. Fold into a burrito and serve warm.

Note: I usually use plant-based cheddar, but every now and then I splurge and use cheese.

Taura: Now, about Quiana. Quiana is my Brostie's wife. You should know me by now. I love creating my own compound words, and

Brostie is Brother + Bestie. Charles Kelley is my Brostie and Quiana is now my Sistie. She has become a sister, a confidant, and someone I truly respect, love, and adore. And she is easily the healthiest person I know.

A few years ago, we all went camping, and believe it or not, it was my first time. I made a big pot of seafood pasta in a garlic-white wine sauce for dinner, and it was amazing, but it did not hold a candle to the simple breakfast burrito Quiana made the next morning. That burrito stayed with me! I remixed it a little to work within my lifestyle rebrand, and I eat it at least once a week. You will too. Pair it with a side of arugula, or add it to your burrito, if you like.

Farmers Market Frittata

Serves 4

Ingredients

- 3 eggs whites
- 3 whole eggs
- ¼ cup unsweetened almond milk or soy milk
- 1 cup spinach, chopped
- 1/3 cup chopped mushrooms of choice
- ½ cup cherry tomatoes, halved
- ½ cup zucchini, diced
- ¼ cup red bell pepper, diced
- ¼ cup red onion, diced
- 2 tbsp olive oil
- ¼ cup plant-based feta or shredded cheese
- Salt and pepper to taste

Directions

1. Preheat oven to 375°F.

2. In a bowl, whisk together eggs, almond milk, salt, and pepper.

3. In a skillet, heat olive oil and sauté zucchini, peppers, and onion until softened. Add spinach and cook until wilted.

4. Pour the egg mixture over the vegetables. Stir gently, then top with tomatoes and plant-based cheese.

5. Bake for 20–25 minutes until set. Slice and serve warm.

Breakfast Sandwich with Plant-Based Sausage

Serves 1

Ingredients

- 1 whole-grain English muffin or healthier biscuit (see recipe below)
- 1 plant-based sausage patty (store-bought or homemade)
- 1 egg or egg substitute, over medium.
- 1 slice plant-based cheddar (or regular, if preferred)
- 1–2 slices tomato or avocado (optional)

Directions

1. Toast an English muffin or a biscuit until golden.

2. Cook plant-based sausage patties according to package instructions or a homemade recipe.

3. Assemble the sandwich: bottom half of muffin, sausage, egg, cheese, and optional toppings. Place the top half on and serve warm.

Note: You can make this as healthy as you'd like. I love using spinach and mushrooms instead of meat, and I almost always use Sola Bagels (low-car/high-fiber) for the bread. I also top the bread with Benecol Light Buttery Spread.

Buttermilk Protein Biscuits

Serves 8 (about 8 biscuits)

Yvonne

When I moved to California, I brought my Southern kitchen with me. I used to make biscuits or corn fritters just about every weekend. Whenever I went home to Alabama, I would bring back Alaga cane syrup. Nothing about those dishes was healthy, but they were full of love. This updated biscuit keeps that same comfort while adding a gentle boost of protein. The texture stays tender, the flavor stays true, and the biscuit still feels like home.

Ingredients

- 2 cups almond flour
- 1/4 cup unflavored whey protein isolate
- 2 tsp baking powder
- 1/2 tsp baking soda
- 1/2 tsp salt
- 2 tbsp coconut oil or olive oil, chilled
- 2 eggs, lightly beaten
- 1/4 cup unsweetened almond milk plus 1 tsp apple cider vinegar (buttermilk substitute)

Directions

1. Preheat oven to 350°F and line a baking sheet with parchment paper.

2. In a medium bowl, mix almond flour, whey protein, baking powder, baking soda, and salt.

3. Cut in the chilled coconut oil until the mixture resembles coarse crumbs.

4. In a separate bowl, whisk the eggs and almond milk–vinegar mixture.

5. Stir the wet mixture into the dry ingredients just until combined. If the dough feels a little dry, add 1 tablespoon almond milk.

6. Drop dough by spoonfuls onto the baking sheet.

7. Bake 15 to 18 minutes, until the biscuits are lightly golden on top.

Notes

Whey isolate adds protein without altering the biscuit's texture. For a dairy-free option, use 1/3 cup plant protein and add 1 to 2 extra tablespoons of almond milk if needed.

Green Godis'

A celebration of everything bright, fresh, and grown from God's green earth. These dishes bring color, crunch, comfort, and creativity to your plate. Some are old family staples, some are inspired by Alabama or California, and others are simple ways to eat more of what supports long-term health. Every dish is a reminder that God is good.

Farmer's Market Salad with Tanecia's Homemade Dressing

Serves 4

Ingredients

- 6 cups mixed seasonal greens
- 1 cucumber, sliced
- 1 cup cherry tomatoes, halved
- 1 red bell pepper, sliced
- ½ cup shredded carrots
- ¼ cup red onion, thinly sliced

Dressing

- 1/3 cup olive oil
- 2 tbsp fresh squeezed lemon juice
- 1 tsp Dijon mustard
- 1 tsp honey or monk fruit

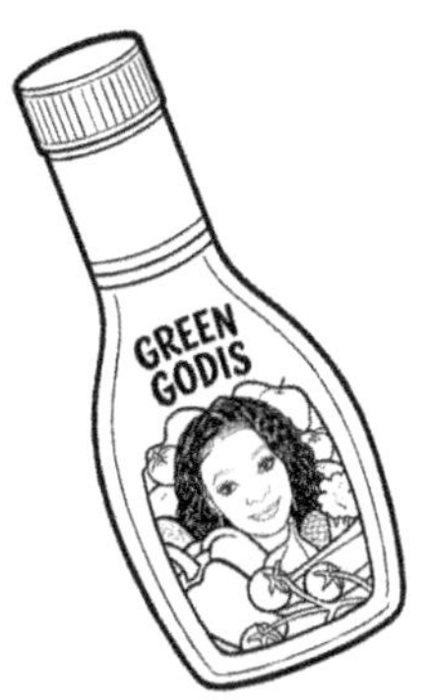

- 2 cloves garlic, minced
- ½ tsp dried thyme
- ½ tsp dried tarragon
- ½ tsp dried oregano
- ½ tsp lemon pepper

Directions

1. Combine salad ingredients in a large bowl.

2. In a jar, shake dressing ingredients until well blended.

3. Pour over salad and toss to coat.

About Tanecia Stinson: (Taura) Tanecia is my younger sister and one of the greatest cooks in the world. She grew up watching me and her mom cook, while also learning from our dad, a true master of barbecue and gumbo. From there, she moved from helping to quietly taking the lead, like a Michelin-star chef in her own right. When she became a mom to my brilliant and handsome nephew Xzavier, another one of my favorite humans to ever walk this beautiful planet, her cooking got even better, and this dressing was born.

It is the kind of recipe you make a double batch of and keep in the fridge, reaching for it again and again. Truly, it is the gift of again and again. It reflects how she balances work and life so beautifully, feeding her family with nourishment, joy, and loads of style.

She also makes what might be the best French toast known to womankind, but I felt her insanely delicious salad dressing belonged here. It is simple, thoughtful, and unforgettable, just like her.

SoCal Kale

Serves 4 to 6

Ingredients

- 2 tbsp ghee
- 2 shallots, minced
- 2 tsp coconut aminos
- ½ tsp mild Dijon mustard
- 1 tsp low sodium chicken Better Than Bouillon
- 3 bunches kale, washed and chopped
- Salt and black pepper

Directions

1. Melt ghee in a skillet over medium heat.

2. Add shallots and cook until translucent.

3. Stir in coconut aminos, mustard, and bouillon.

4. Add kale in batches and cook until wilted but still crunchy.

5. Season with salt and black pepper.

Mom's Succotash

Serves 6

Ingredients

- 1 tbsp unsalted butter
- 1 tbsp olive oil
- 3 cloves garlic, minced
- 1 cup onion, diced
- 1 cup okra, sliced
- 2 cups lima beans
- 2 cups fresh corn
- 1 red bell pepper, diced
- 2 Roma tomatoes, diced
- 1 tsp vegetable Better Than Bouillon
- 1 tsp smoked paprika
- ½ tsp thyme
- ½ tsp black pepper
- ½ tsp salt
- Juice of ½ lemon

Directions

1. Heat butter and oil in a skillet over medium heat.

2. Add garlic and onion. Cook until softened.

3. Add okra, lima beans, and corn to the bouillon. Cook for 8 to 10 minutes.

4. Add the bell pepper, tomatoes, and seasonings. Cook for 3 to 4 minutes.

5. Finish with lemon juice.

Date Night Brussels Sprouts

Serves 4

Ingredients

- 1 lb Brussels sprouts, halved
- 1 tbsp avocado oil
- 2 cloves garlic, minced
- ¼ cup dried cranberries
- ¼ cup chopped almonds
- 2 tbsp fresh dill
- 2 tbsp fresh mint
- 2 tbsp olive oil
- Juice of ½ lemon
- ½ cup whipped Greek yogurt
- Coarse salt

Directions

1. Preheat air fryer to 375°F.

2. Toss Brussels sprouts with avocado oil and cook 12 to 15 minutes.

3. Toss hot sprouts with garlic, cranberries, and almonds.

4. Whisk dill, mint, olive oil, lemon, and salt.

5. Spread the whipped yogurt on a plate and pile the sprouts on top. Drizzle with the herb dressing.

Carol Ware's Heavenly Tomatoes

Preheat oven to 400 degrees

Ingredients

- 2 packages of Heavenly San Marzano Tomatoes
- (Purchase @ Trader Joe's)

USE SMALL CHERRY TOMATOES AS A SUBSTITUTE

- Slice in half
- 3 to 4 cloves fresh garlic
- Sliced lengthwise
- Fresh basil
- Gather a bunch of leaves and chop or tear leaves
- Fresh Italian parsley
- Tear a bunch and chop finely

Extra Virgin Olive Oil

- Kosher salt
- Black pepper
- Red pepper flakes

Instructions

Spread olive oil onto a sheet pan.

Place tomato halves flesh side down onto the pan.

Sprinkle garlic over tomatoes as evenly as possible.

Sprinkle basil and parsley evenly over tomatoes.

Drizzle Extra Virgin Olive Oil over tomatoes.

Add salt and pepper over the top and sprinkle red pepper flakes sparingly.

Place in preheated oven and roast for 20 to 25 minutes.

Remove from oven and, using a fork, mash the tomatoes. Place back in the oven to absorb tomato juices and form the "caviar."

Prepare thin slices of baguette. Sprinkle with Extra Virgin Olive Oil and place in oven briefly to warm or toast.

Place tomato "caviar" in a bowl and serve with baguette slices on the side.

About Carol Ware: (Taura) I met Carol and Leon Ware soon after moving to Los Angeles around 2004. We folded into being family right away and adopted each other as our own. I was a big fan of Leon long before meeting him. He was a legendary songwriter, having written hits like *I WANNA BE WHERE YOU ARE*, the entire Marvin Gaye *I WANT YOU* album, and some of my favorite Minnie Riperton songs.

Their home was always filled with love and the best food, because Carol could make the simplest things taste so good. One of my favorites is these tomatoes, but you have to be careful or you can easily eat a full baguette with them. I also love them alongside Mediterranean food, and they are just as delicious.

Carol is a wonderful storyteller and someone that I lovingly call my "SoCal Mom". She has shared so many beautiful memories over the years that have become life lessons for me. We have been extended family all of these years, and I am so grateful that she shared her famous tomato recipe with me.

Shredded Brussels Sprouts Salad

Serves 4

Ingredients

- 3 cups shaved Brussels sprouts
- 2 tbsp olive oil
- Juice of ½ lemon
- ¼ cup dried cherries
- ¼ cup toasted walnuts
- ¼ cup feta or plant based cheese
- Salt and black pepper

Directions

1. Toss all ingredients together.

2. Serve chilled or at room temperature.

Cauliflower and Potato Mash

Serves 4

Ingredients

- 1 medium head cauliflower, cut into florets
- 1 large Yukon Gold potato, peeled and cubed
- ¼ cup Greek yogurt
- 2 teaspoons nutritional yeast
- 1 tablespoon plant-based butter
- 1 tablespoon olive oil
- 2 cloves garlic, minced
- Salt and black pepper
- Optional: fresh chives

Directions

1. Boil the cauliflower and potato in salted water until tender.

2. Drain well.

3. Mash or blend with Greek yogurt, nutritional yeast, plant-based butter, olive oil, garlic, salt, and black pepper.

4. Sprinkle with fresh chives if you like.

Mother McElhaney's Glazed Carrots

Ingredients

- 1 lb fresh carrots (3-4 large carrots)
- 3-4 Tablespoons butter
- 1/4 – 1/2 cup brown sugar, enough glaze to cover the carrots
- 1/4 – 1/2 cup fresh-squeezed lemon juice
- pinch of salt

Directions

1. Pre-heat oven to 375.

2. Clean, peel, and half carrots, cut into sticks.

3. Add carrots to a saucepan; Parboil carrots until al dente (should still be firm to the fork test because they will continue cooking at the next step)

4. While the carrots boil, make your glaze.

5. Add lemon juice to brown sugar to make a brown sugar syrup.

6. Drain carrots and place in a medium loaf pan

7. Melt butter atop the hot carrots. Stir gentle to cover.

8. Pour the glaze atop the carrots. Glaze should cover/touch all/ most carrots

9. Bake for 10-15 minutes until tender and the sauce has thickened.

About Mother McElhaney: (Yvonne) I call her MizMac, but my heart calls her Mom. She is the mother of Clarence, who shared his stroke journey earlier, and of four other incredible children, including my late best friend, Chauming. We called her Charm, but my heart called her sister.

One of my earliest memories after meeting Charm was being invited to a big McElhaney family dinner. This was no ordinary soul food spread. Everything was vegetable-forward, clean, and nourishing. Maybe that is why, even in her late eighties, Mother McElhaney has the skin of someone half her age. She is also deeply healthy where it truly counts, on the inside. Somehow, she manages this while still enjoying her chocolate, a reminder that care, balance, and joy can live beautifully side by side.

Both Taura and I love cooked carrots, but raw carrots were not so much our thing until we tried Mrs. Barbara McElhaney's glazed carrots. They are not too sweet, just savory enough, and have a delicious, distinctive flavor. Mhhm mmh mmh.

Blistered Shishito Peppers with Lime Salt

Serves 4

Ingredients

- 3 cups shishito peppers
- 1 tbsp olive oil
- Juice of ½ lime
- Sea salt

Directions

1. Heat a skillet over medium–high heat.

2. Add peppers and let them blister.

3. Drizzle with olive oil.

4. Finish with lime juice and sea salt.

California Kimchi

A light, bright, no-heat version inspired by California wellness kitchens.
Serves 6

Ingredients

- 3 cups Napa cabbage, chopped
- 1 cup shredded carrots
- 1 cup thinly sliced Persian cucumbers
- 2 green onions, sliced
- 1 clove garlic, minced
- 1 tsp grated ginger
- 1½ tsp salt
- Juice of ½ lemon
- ½ tsp dried oregano or thyme

Directions

1. Combine cabbage, carrots, cucumbers, and green onions in a bowl.

2. Add salt and massage for 3 to 5 minutes until the vegetables soften and release liquid.

3. Add garlic, ginger, lemon juice, and herbs.

4. Pack tightly into a jar, pressing down to keep vegetables submerged under the liquid.

5. Cover loosely and ferment at room temperature for 1 to 2 days.

6. Refrigerate once lightly tangy.

Green Godis Wrap-Up

Below are simple ways to add more fresh food to your daily routine. These are quick, flexible ideas you can make without a recipe and adjust to your taste.

Arugula and Tomato Salad

Arugula, sliced Roma tomatoes, olives, parsley, and a sprinkle of feta. Drizzle with olive oil and lemon juice. Season with cracked black pepper.

Broccoli with Garlic Sauce

Steam or roast the broccoli. Toss with a quick sauce made from olive oil, minced garlic, lemon, and salt. Add tofu or chicken for extra protein.

Cucumber with Vinegar and Thyme

Slice the cucumbers thin. Add a splash of vinegar, a pinch of salt, and a sprinkle of dried thyme. Chill before serving.

Simple Vegetable Stir Fry

Sauté any mix of vegetables in olive oil with garlic and a little tamari or coconut aminos. Serve alone or over quinoa or brown rice.

Garlicky Lemon Greens

Any greens you have on hand, lightly sautéed in olive oil with garlic and lemon juice. Salt to taste. (optional: I also top with fresh parsley and more lemon)

Sautéed Mushrooms, Onions, and Zucchini

Cook sliced mushrooms, onions, and zucchini in olive oil until tender. Season with salt, black pepper, and a little thyme. Serve warm as a side dish or over grains.

Quick Roasted Veggie Plate

Roast whatever vegetables you have with olive oil, salt, and pepper. Serve with a spoonful of hummus on the side.

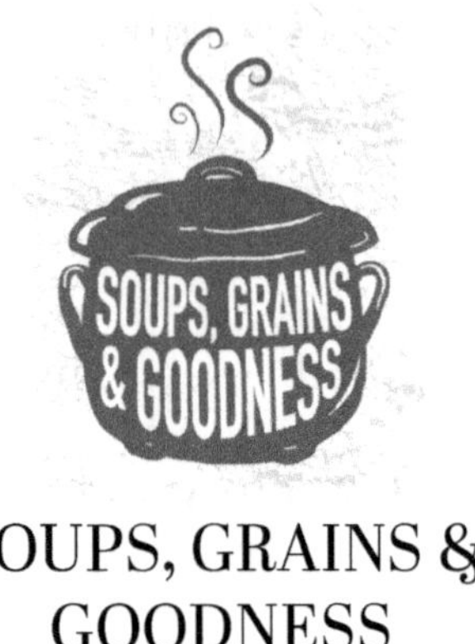

SOUPS, GRAINS &
GOODNESS

Soups, Grains and Goodness

You can always find my mom in the soup and salad section, especially during the fall or winter, and I haven't met a pasta dish I didn't like. But in this chapter, the goal is to make simple sides and lighter bowls feel like main characters. We will lean on Carbe Diem and other low-carb pasta options, a few grains and legumes, and dishes that come together easily. We will also end this section with easy restaurant-style bowls made from leftovers and whatever you already have in your fridge.

Plant Based Broccoli Cheddar Style Soup

Ingredients

- 1 tbsp olive oil
- 1 cup onion, diced
- 3 cloves garlic, minced
- 4 cups broccoli florets
- 1 cup carrots, diced
- 3 cups low sodium vegetable broth
- 1 cup raw cashews, soaked and drained
- ½ cup nutritional yeast
- 1 cup unsweetened almond milk

- 1 tsp turmeric
- ½ tsp smoked paprika
- Salt and black pepper to taste

Directions

Heat olive oil in a pot over medium heat. Add onion and garlic and cook until softened. Add broccoli, carrots, and broth. Simmer until the vegetables are tender. Blend soaked cashews, nutritional yeast, almond milk, turmeric, and paprika until creamy. Stir into the pot and simmer a few more minutes. Season with salt and pepper and serve warm.

Reset Vegetable Soup with Cabbage and Spinach

Ingredients

- 1 tbsp olive oil
- 1 cup onion, diced
- 1 cup celery, sliced
- 1 cup carrots, diced
- 3 cloves garlic, minced
- 3 cups cabbage, chopped
- 1 zucchini, diced
- 6 cups low-sodium vegetable broth
- 2 cups spinach
- Salt and black pepper to taste
- Fresh herbs and lemon to finish

Directions

Heat olive oil in a large pot and sauté the onion, celery, and carrots until softened. Add the garlic, cabbage, and zucchini. Pour in the broth and simmer until the vegetables are tender. Stir in the spinach and cook briefly until wilted. Season with salt, black pepper, fresh herbs, and a squeeze of lemon.

Black Bean Chili

Ingredients

- 1 tbsp olive oil
- 1 cup onion, diced
- 1 cup bell pepper, diced
- 3 cloves garlic, minced
- 2 cans black beans, drained
- 1 can diced tomatoes
- 1 to 1½ cups broth
- 1 tbsp chili powder
- 1 tsp cumin
- ½ tsp smoked paprika
- ½ cup tomato sauce (optional for a smoother texture)
- Salt and black pepper to taste
- Lime and cilantro to finish

Directions

Sauté the onion, bell pepper, and garlic in olive oil until softened. Add the black beans, diced tomatoes, broth, chili powder, cumin, and smoked paprika. For a smoother, less chunky chili, stir in tomato sauce or mash a small portion of the beans before simmering. Let the chili cook until thick and flavorful. Finish with lime and cilantro.

Simple Stir-Fry with Vegetables

Ingredients

- 1 tbsp avocado oil
- 3 cups mixed vegetables such as broccoli, zucchini, mushrooms, carrots, or cabbage
- 3 cloves garlic, minced
- 1 to 2 tbsp coconut aminos
- Splash of rice vinegar
- Salt and black pepper

Directions

Heat avocado oil in a skillet and cook vegetables until tender but still crisp. Add garlic, coconut aminos, and rice vinegar. Toss until coated. Serve over grains or cauliflower rice.

Tomato Braised Lentils

Ingredients

- 1 tbsp olive oil
- 1 cup onion, diced
- 3 cloves garlic, minced
- 1½ cups dried lentils, rinsed
- 1 cup cherry or grape tomatoes, halved
- 1 can crushed tomatoes
- 2 cups low sodium broth
- 1 tbsp chicken Better Than Bouillon
- 1 tsp dried oregano
- ½ tsp smoked paprika
- ¼ tsp turmeric
- ½ tsp onion powder
- ½ tsp garlic powder
- 2 tbsp balsamic vinegar or fresh lemon juice
- Salt and black pepper to taste
- Fresh parsley or basil, chopped

Directions

Heat the olive oil in a pot over medium heat. Add the onion and sauté until softened. Stir in the garlic and cook for one more minute. Add the cherry tomatoes and cook, stirring occasionally, until they soften and begin to burst, releasing their juices.

Stir in the lentils, crushed tomatoes, broth, Better Than Bouillon, oregano, smoked paprika, turmeric, onion powder, and garlic powder. Cover and simmer until the lentils are tender and the tomatoes are fully incorporated into the sauce.

Finish by stirring in balsamic vinegar or lemon juice. Season with salt and black pepper to taste, then fold in fresh herbs just before serving. Serve with rice, or quinoa, or in wrap, or with pita chips…or as a soup base…the sky is the limit.

p.s. people will ask you to make these lentils for every function.

Barley with Mushrooms, Shallots and White Wine

Ingredients

- 1 tbsp olive oil
- 2 shallots, thinly sliced
- 3 cups mushrooms, sliced
- 2 cloves garlic, minced
- 1 cup pearled barley, rinsed
- ½ cup dry white wine
- 3 cups low sodium broth
- 1 tsp thyme
- Salt and black pepper to taste
- Fresh parsley, chopped (for finishing)

Directions

Heat the olive oil in a pot over medium heat. Add the sliced shallots and cook until softened. Stir in the mushrooms and cook until they brown. Add the garlic and cook for a few seconds until fragrant. Add the barley and stir to coat it with the aromatics. Pour in the white wine and cook until most of it evaporates. Add the broth and thyme. Bring to a simmer, cover, and cook until the barley is tender and most of the liquid has been absorbed. Season with salt and black pepper. Finish with fresh parsley.

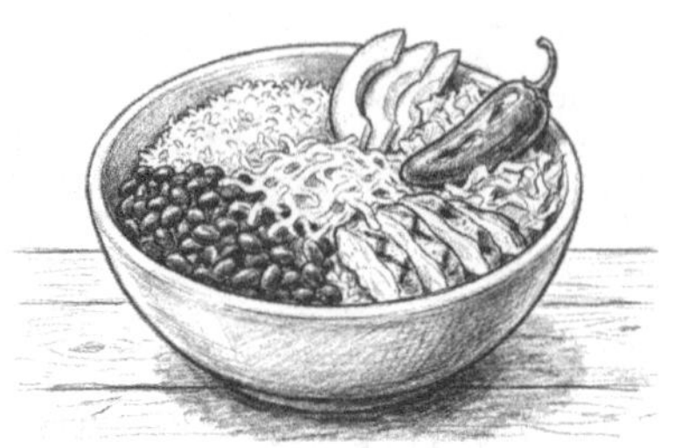

THE BOWL CUT

Mediterranean Tuna or Sardine Bowl

Add cooked quinoa to a bowl, then top with tuna or sardines, sliced cucumber, cherry tomatoes, olives, capers, and red onion. Drizzle with olive oil and lemon juice. A light seasoning is all it needs.

Mexican-Inspired Bowl

Start with warm quinoa or brown rice, then layer black beans, roasted corn, salsa, and sliced avocado. Add a spoonful of Greek yogurt or plant-based yogurt, then finish with cilantro and lime. Leftover chicken, shrimp, or tofu fit right in.

California Clean Out the Fridge Bowl

Add fresh greens to a bowl, then top with leftover roasted vegetables. Add quinoa or lentils. Finish with tahini or hummus, lemon juice, salt, and pepper.

Warm Stir-Fry Bowl

Add cooked quinoa or cauliflower rice to a bowl, then top with leftover stir-fried vegetables. Add a fried or poached egg and a splash of soy sauce, coconut aminos, or rice vinegar.

Simple Italian Bowl

Toss cooked Carbe Diem pasta with roasted broccoli or zucchini. Add quinoa for extra fiber. Drizzle with olive oil, sprinkle with Parmesan or nutritional yeast, and add herbs.

Warm Lentil and Egg Bowl

Spoon tomato braised lentils into a bowl and top with a soft boiled or jammy egg. Add a handful of arugula or spinach and finish with olive oil, salt, and black pepper. Simple, filling, and deeply comforting.

Middle Eastern Inspired Bowl
Start with warm lentils or quinoa. Add chopped cucumber, tomato, and red onion. Finish with a dollop of hummus or labneh, olive oil, lemon juice, and fresh parsley.

Soul Bowl
Start with warm brown rice. Add red beans, roasted or air-fried sweet potatoes, and diced air fried chicken. Finish with olive oil, salt, black pepper, and a splash of hot sauce.

Sushi Brown Rice Bowl
Start with warm brown rice. Add raw or seared salmon or tofu, sliced cucumber, avocado, and shredded carrot. Finish with soy sauce or coconut aminos, a splash of rice vinegar, and a sprinkle of sesame seeds. Optional nori snacks on the side.

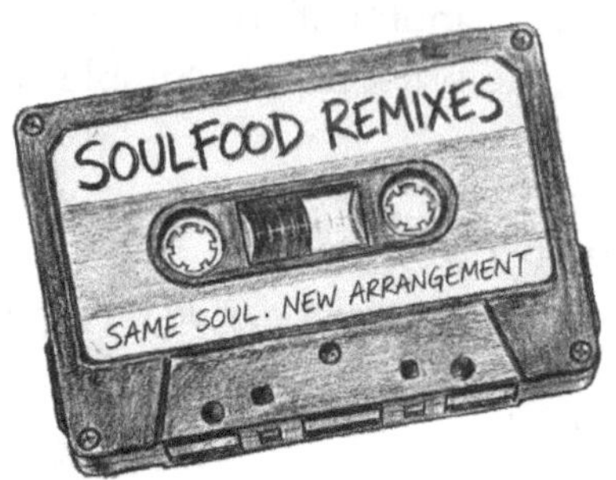

Same Soul,
New Arrangement Soulfood Remixes

Yvonne

The food I grew up on had a rhythm of its own. My mother, Mittie Lee Morton, cooked by instinct. She didn't measure, she didn't read recipes, and she didn't need to. She fed us from memory and from her heart, and the dishes she made were full of comfort, history, and soul. I passed those recipes down to Taura the same way, but as life changed, so did our understanding of what our bodies needed. We still love the same flavors, but we had to learn how to prepare them in ways that support the season we are in now.

Taura

I never want to lose the story in the food I grew up loving. I just want to enjoy it without feeling like I'm fighting my own body afterward. These recipes are not about restriction. They are about arrangement. The same songs, the same melodies, but written in a key that fits where we are today. We took the dishes that shaped us and learned how to make them lighter, cleaner, and more supportive without losing the soul that made them unforgettable.

Together

These dishes are meant to be enjoyed in moderation, but they are healthier alternatives to the celebratory meals that have graced our tables for generations. This is how we honor where we come from while protecting where we are going. The same soul, arranged for a new season.

Cornless' Bread

Taura

Cornbread and collard greens will always be among my favorite meals. Before I learned to braise my greens, I smothered them in hot sauce and cooked them until there was no life left in them. Somewhere along the way, I realized my cornbread needed a remix, too. Since I watch my carbs, I came up with this Cornless Bread. It is so good you will not miss the corn. And if jalapeño is not your thing, just leave it out. But honestly, who needs hot sauce when you have the pepper?

Ingredients

- 5 cups blanched almond flour
- 1 tablespoon baking powder
- 1/3 cup monk fruit sugar
- 1 teaspoon sea salt
- 2/3 cup Benecol, melted, plus more for greasing
- 2/3 cup unsweetened almond milk
- 3 large eggs
- 3 flax eggs
- 1 tablespoon sweet corn extract
- 1/3 cup fresh or canned corn
- 1 small onion, minced
- 1 jalapeño, minced

Instructions

Preheat oven to 350°F. Grease a 9x13-inch pan with Benecol. Whisk together the dry ingredients in one bowl and the wet ingredients in another. Combine, fold in the vegetables, and bake for 30 to 35 minutes until golden.

Cornless' Bread Dressin'

Ingredients

- 1 batch Cornless' Bread, cooled and crumbled
- 2 tablespoons vegan butter or Benecol
- 1 medium onion, finely diced
- 2 celery stalks, finely diced
- 1 small green bell pepper, chopped
- 1½ cups vegetable broth
- 2 eggs or flax eggs
- 1 teaspoon poultry seasoning
- 1 teaspoon garlic powder
- ½ teaspoon black pepper
- ½ teaspoon salt
- ½ teaspoon dried sage
- ½ cup fresh parsley
- 2 tablespoons fresh thyme
- 2 tablespoons fresh sage
- 1 tablespoon plant based butter
- 1 teaspoon olive oil
- Low carb breadcrumbs (optional)

Directions

Sauté the fresh sage in butter and olive oil. Add the onion, celery, and bell pepper and cook until softened. Combine with the crumbled

Cornless' Bread, dried sage, herbs, eggs, and broth. Bake at 375°F for 30 to 35 minutes, until set.

Tip
Low-carb breads like Sola or Hero make excellent homemade breadcrumbs.

Auntie Von's Candied Yams

Ingredients

- 4 to 5 yams, sliced
- ½ cup plant based butter
- ¼ cup brown monk fruit sweetener
- ¼ cup white monk fruit sweetener
- ¼ cup maple syrup or agave
- 1 teaspoon vanilla
- 1 teaspoon cinnamon
- ½ teaspoon nutmeg
- ¼ teaspoon salt
- 1 teaspoon lemon juice (optional)

Directions

Melt the butter with sweeteners, maple syrup, vanilla, cinnamon, nutmeg, salt, and lemon juice. Layer in the yams, coat them in syrup, cover, and cook 45 minutes to 1 hour on low. Spoon syrup over the yams every 15 minutes until glossy and tender.

Mac & Cheese Made Lighter

Ingredients

- 2 cups Carbe Diem or high fiber pasta
- 1 cup raw cashews, soaked
- 1 cup almond or oat milk
- 1 cup shredded cheddar or plant based cheddar
- ¼ cup nutritional yeast
- 2 tablespoons butter or plant-based butter
- 1 tablespoon garlic powder
- 1 tablespoon onion powder
- ½ teaspoon smoked paprika
- Salt and black pepper
- Extra cheese for topping

Directions

Blend cashews with milk. Heat in a pot with cheese, butter, nutritional yeast, and seasonings until smooth. Fold in cooked pasta. Top with cheese and bake or broil until browned.

Healthy Southern Collards

Ingredients

- 1 tablespoon olive oil
- 1 cup onion, diced
- 3 cloves garlic, minced
- 8 cups collard greens, cleaned and sliced
- 3 to 4 cups broth (vegetable or chicken)
- 1 teaspoon smoked paprika
- 1 teaspoon Better Than Bouillon vegetable base **or** 1 small smoked turkey wing
- ½ teaspoon garlic powder
- ½ teaspoon onion powder
- 1 tablespoon apple cider vinegar
- Salt and black pepper to taste
- Optional: a pinch of crushed red pepper, a splash of hot sauce, or ½ teaspoon brown sugar for balance

Directions

Clean your greens thoroughly and remove the thick stems. Heat the olive oil in a large pot over medium heat. Add the diced onion and sauté until soft. Stir in the garlic and cook until fragrant. Add the collard greens in batches, allowing them to wilt. Pour in the broth, smoked paprika, vegetable base or turkey wing, garlic powder, and onion powder. Stir well. Bring to a simmer, reduce the heat, cover, and cook until the greens are tender and the broth is rich with flavor. Finish with apple cider vinegar and adjust the seasoning with salt, black pepper, and optional heat or sweetness. Simmer a few minutes longer before serving.

Special Note
Stir-fried lemony garlic greens are a fast, delicious alternative. Thinly slice your cleaned collards and sauté them over medium-high heat with olive oil, garlic, a squeeze of fresh lemon, sea salt, and black pepper. They are bright, tender, and ready in 15 minutes.

Crispy Air-Fried Chicken Wings

Serves 4

Ingredients

- 2 to 3 pounds chicken wings
- 2 tablespoons cornstarch
- 1 tablespoon olive oil
- 1 tablespoon garlic powder
- 1 tablespoon onion powder
- 1 teaspoon smoked paprika
- 1 teaspoon dried thyme
- 1 teaspoon dried oregano
- 1/2 teaspoon turmeric
- 1/2 teaspoon ground mustard
- Salt and black pepper
- Avocado oil spray

Directions

- Pat chicken wings dry.
- Place wings in a bowl and toss with olive oil.
- In a separate bowl, mix cornstarch, garlic powder, onion powder, smoked paprika, thyme, oregano, turmeric, ground mustard, salt, and black pepper.
- Coat wings evenly with the seasoning mixture.
- Lightly spray wings with avocado oil spray.

- Place wings in the air fryer basket in a single layer.
- Air fry at 390°F for 22 to 26 minutes, shaking halfway, until crisp and golden.
- Serve immediately or toss with your preferred sauce.

Air Fried Fish

Serves 4

Ingredients

- 4 fish fillets
- 1 tablespoon olive oil
- 1/3 cup fine cornmeal
- 2 tablespoons cornstarch
- 2 teaspoons garlic powder
- 2 teaspoons onion powder
- 1 teaspoon smoked paprika
- 1/2 teaspoon dried thyme
- 1 teaspoon seasoning salt
- Black pepper
- 1 egg, beaten
- Avocado oil spray
- Fresh parsley
- Lemon wedges

Directions

- Pat the fish dry and lightly rub with olive oil.
- In a large bag, combine cornmeal, cornstarch, garlic powder, onion powder, smoked paprika, dried thyme, seasoning salt, and black pepper. Shake well to mix.

- Dip each fillet into the beaten egg, then place it in the bag. Shake until well coated.

- Spray both sides of the fish with avocado oil spray.

- Preheat the air fryer to 400°F.

- Place the coated fillets in a single layer in the air fryer basket without stacking or overlapping.

- Air fry for 8 to 12 minutes, depending on thickness, turning once if preferred, until crisp and golden.

- Top with fresh parsley and lemon before serving.

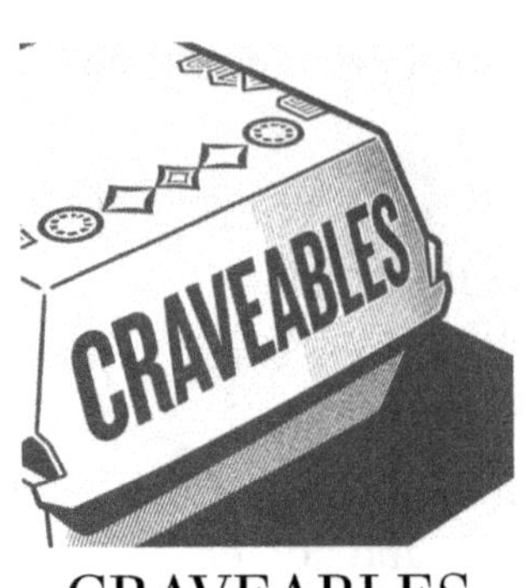

CRAVEABLES

Taura

If you are like me, you crave things, and the next thing you know, you are ten pounds heavier. My rule of thumb is to make it at home, make it delicious, and make it healthy. I don't eat these dishes daily, but once a week gives me the fix I crave without tipping the scale. These are the things I love, remixed to satisfy the craving while keeping me aligned with my goals.

Rich Girl Po' Boy Remix

Not a Po' Boy, but rich in health of body, mind, and soul. Lightly bread shrimp by dipping in beaten egg, then into cornstarch mixed with Cajun seasoning, garlic powder, onion powder, and salt. Air-fry until crisp. Make a healthier remoulade with Greek yogurt, Dijon mustard, chopped pickles, smoked paprika or Cajun seasoning, lemon juice, and a pinch of monk fruit sugar. Layer shrimp on toasted low-carb bread or a low-carb bagel with shredded lettuce, tomato, and extra pickles.

Banh Mi Bagel

Toast a low-carb bagel. Mix Greek yogurt with rice vinegar, minced garlic, monk fruit sugar, and chili flakes, then spread a thin layer over the bread. Add air-fried chicken or shrimp, pickled carrots and daikon, thin cucumber slices, cilantro, and jalapeño. Finish with lime for brightness and crunch.

Lemon Pepper Wing Remix

Season wings with garlic powder, onion powder, a pinch of salt, and a little olive oil. Air-fry until crisp. Toss with warm lemon juice, lemon pepper seasoning, olive oil, and a tiny pinch of monk fruit sugar. Serve immediately.

Pizza Wrap Remix

Spread marinara on a low-carb wrap, then top with mozzarella, veggies or turkey pepperoni, and Italian seasoning. Air-fry or toast until the edges crisp and the cheese melts. Slice and enjoy a lighter pizza moment.

BBQ Chicken Pizza Remix

Spread low-sugar BBQ sauce on a low-carb tortilla. Add shredded chicken, thinly sliced red onion, and mozzarella or plant-based cheese. Air-fry or bake until bubbly and crisp. Finish with cilantro.

Crispy Burrito Remix

Fill a low-carb wrap with seasoned turkey or beans, sautéed peppers and onions, and Greek yogurt instead of sour cream, along with a little plant-based or low-fat cheese. Fold tightly and air-fry until golden brown. Serve with salsa or hot sauce.

Shrimp & Grits Remix (Cauliflower Edition)

Pulse steamed cauliflower until it resembles grits, then warm it with almond milk, garlic powder, onion powder, a spoonful of nutritional yeast or light cheese, and a little Benecol or plant-based butter. Sauté shrimp with garlic, diced tomato, parsley, thyme, smoked paprika, and a spoonful of Greek yogurt. Finish with lemon and spoon everything over the cauliflower grits.

Taco Tuesday

Use Mission 25-calorie tortillas or A La Madre tortillas, lightly spray with olive oil, and air-fry until crisp but still flexible. Fill with slow-cooker chicken seasoned with cumin, garlic, onion powder, chili powder, and lime, or plant-based beef cooked with taco seasoning. Top with lettuce, tomato, or jalapeños. Make the sauce by mixing Greek yogurt, taco seasoning, and a squeeze of lime.

Tuna Melt

Combine canned tuna with Greek yogurt, Dijon mustard, celery, red onion, lemon, and dill. Spoon onto low-carb bread, top with cheese, and air-fry until bubbly and golden. Add a tomato or avocado to elevate the flavor.

ABJ Remix (Grilled Almond Butter & Jelly)

Spread almond butter and no-sugar-added jelly on low-carb bread. Lightly spray the outside and grill or air-fry until warm and golden. It delivers classic comfort without excess sugar.

Chicken Strips with Sugar-Free Hunni Mustard Remix

Slice chicken breasts into strips and season with garlic powder, onion powder, smoked paprika, salt, and pepper. Dip in beaten egg, then into almond flour mixed with a little cornstarch for crunch. Air-fry until golden. Make the dipping sauce by mixing a sugar-free honey alternative with Dijon mustard, a squeeze of lemon, and a pinch of monk fruit sugar for balance. Serve hot for the perfect sweet-savory bite.

Mickey Deez Chicken Wrap Remix

Use a low-carb tortilla and fill it with air-fried chicken or shrimp, shredded lettuce, a sprinkle of low-fat cheese, and a drizzle of light ranch. Wrap it tightly and air-fry for a minute or two to warm it through. It feels like drive-thru comfort, remixed for real life.

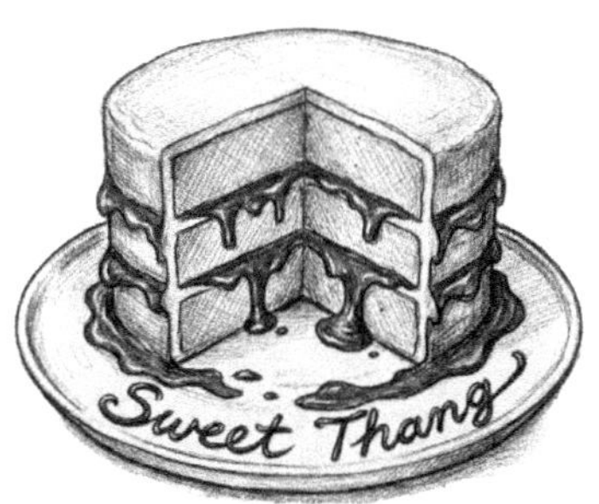

Oh, Sweet Thang.

Yvonne: I am known for my Red Velvet Cake. I first made it in 1976, using a recipe passed down to me by Mr. Lothlen, the father of my former brother-in-law. When he passed, the torch landed in my hands, and I've carried it ever since. I've made this cake for everyone from soul legends Raphael Saadiq and Anthony Hamilton to beauty mogul Damone Roberts and his husband Ramone. In fact, Ramone once stood in the bathroom eating the very last cupcake after I baked them their own batch…sharing is always caring with those two, but not that day. (chuckle)

Taura doesn't eat Red Velvet at all, and I only taste it every now and again. I think it's because we've smelled, packaged, and tasted it so many times over the years that the craving faded. But we know how beloved this cake is and how powerful sugar can be. While people should absolutely indulge from time to time, some folks need stronger guardrails. That's what this version is…guardrails for anyone who has non-negotiables around sugar. And I must say, the no-added-sugar version is just as tasty, though I still make both upon request.

If you're holding this book, maybe start with this version. Without further ado… Auntie Von's famous Red Velvet Cake, along with a short collection of sweet endings for your new beginnings.

Auntie Von's Red Velvet Cake

Preheat your oven to 350°F. Grease and flour two 9-inch round cake pans and line the bottoms with parchment paper.

CAKE

- 2 - Cups Vegetable Oil
- 2 - Cups Monk Fruit Sugar
- 3 - Large Eggs (Room Temp)
- 2 3/4 - Cups Flour (Plus)
- 3 Tablespoons Corn Starch
- 2 - Teaspoons Unsweetened Cocoa
- 1 1/2 Teaspoons Baking Soda
- 1/2 - Teaspoon Baking Powder
- 1- Teaspoon Salt
- 1 - Cup Buttermilk plus
- 1/4 Cup Whole Milk
- 2- Tablespoons Red Food Color
- 2- Teaspoons White Vinegar
- 2- Tablespoons Vanilla
- 1/2 Teaspoon Lemon Flavor

Cream Cheese Frosting

- 1- 8oz Package Cream Cheese
- 1- Cube Butter
- 1- Box Powdered Sugar

- 3- Teaspoons Vanilla
- 1/2 Teaspoon Lemon

In a large bowl, whisk together the flour, corn starch, cocoa powder, baking soda, baking powder, and salt. Set aside. In a separate small bowl or measuring cup, stir together the buttermilk, whole milk, red food coloring, and white vinegar. Set that aside as well.

In a large mixing bowl, beat together the vegetable oil and monk fruit sugar until well combined. Add the eggs one at a time, beating well after each addition, then mix in the vanilla and lemon flavor.

Gradually alternate adding the dry ingredient mixture and the buttermilk mixture into the wet ingredients, beginning and ending with the dry ingredients. Mix just until everything is combined. Do not overmix.

Divide the batter evenly between your prepared pans and bake at 350°F for 30–35 minutes, or until a toothpick inserted in the center comes out clean. Let the cakes cool in the pans for 10 minutes, then turn them out onto a wire rack and allow to cool completely before frosting.

Cream Cheese Frosting

1 8oz Package Cream Cheese 1 Cube Butter 1 Box Powdered Sugar 3 Teaspoons Vanilla 1/2 Teaspoon Lemon

Make sure your cream cheese and butter are both at room temperature. Beat them together until smooth and fluffy. Add the vanilla and lemon and mix to combine. Gradually add the powdered sugar and beat until the frosting is smooth and creamy.

Once the cake layers are completely cool, place the first layer on your serving plate and spread a generous amount of frosting on top. Set the second layer on top and frost the top and sides of the cake. Refrigerate for at least 30 minutes before slicing for clean, beautiful cuts. Enjoy!

Raw Strawberry Cheesecake

Crust

- 1 cup almonds or pecans
- 1 cup walnuts
- 8–10 Medjool dates
- 1 teaspoon vanilla
- Pinch of salt

Filling

- 2 cups soaked cashews
- 1 cup strawberries
- ¼ cup coconut oil
- ¼ cup almond milk
- 2 tablespoons monk fruit
- 1 teaspoon vanilla

Directions

Blend the crust and press into the pan. Blend the filling until creamy. Spread the filling over the crust and freeze until firm.

Sweet Potato Pie

Ingredients

- 3 large or 4 medium sweet potatoes
- 2 tablespoons coconut oil or avocado oil
- 1 cup salted butter, room temperature
- 1 cup granulated monkfruit sugar
- ½ cup monkfruit brown sugar
- 3 eggs
- 1 tablespoon vanilla bean gel or vanilla bean paste
- ½ teaspoon cinnamon
- ½ teaspoon nutmeg
- ½ teaspoon ground ginger, optional
- 1 can (12 oz) evaporated milk
- 1 unbaked 9 inch pie crust

Whipped Cream Topping

- 1 cup heavy whipping cream
- 2 tablespoons monkfruit powdered sugar
- ½ teaspoon vanilla extract or vanilla bean gel

Directions

Preheat the oven to 400 degrees. Wash the sweet potatoes, rub them with coconut or avocado oil, and roast them on a baking sheet until tender. Let them cool, then scoop the flesh into a bowl and mash until smooth. Lower the oven temperature to 350 degrees.

Cream together the butter, granulated monkfruit sugar, and monkfruit brown sugar. Add the mashed sweet potatoes and mix well. Beat in the eggs, then stir in the vanilla bean gel or paste, cinnamon, nutmeg, and ginger. Slowly mix in the evaporated milk until the filling is smooth.

Pour the filling into the unbaked pie crust and bake for 55 to 65 minutes, until the center is set but still slightly jiggly. Cool completely before slicing.

For the whipped cream, beat the heavy cream, monkfruit powdered sugar, and vanilla to soft peaks. Top each slice with it.

Air Fryer Doughnuts

Ingredients

- 1 cup almond flour
- 2 tablespoons coconut flour
- ¼ cup monk fruit
- 1 teaspoon baking powder
- ¼ teaspoon cinnamon
- 2 eggs
- ¼ cup almond milk
- 2 tablespoons melted Benecol
- 1 teaspoon vanilla

Directions

- Pipe into donut molds and air-fry at 350°F for 8 to 10 minutes until lightly golden.
- Topping Options
- Sugar-free chocolate dip
- Vanilla glaze
- Cinnamon monk fruit dust

Vanilla Bean Nice Cream

Ingredients

- ½ cup full fat cottage cheese
- ½ cup full fat plain Greek yogurt
- 2 to 3 teaspoons monkfruit sweetener
- Seeds from ½ vanilla bean or 1 teaspoon vanilla bean paste
- Pinch of salt
- Optional: 1 teaspoon allulose or 1 tablespoon cream cheese for softer texture

Instructions

Blend all ingredients until completely smooth and glossy. Taste and adjust sweetness. Freeze 2 to 3 hours until scoopable. Let sit 5 minutes before serving.

Strawberry Nice Cream

Ingredients

- ½ cup full fat cottage cheese
- ½ cup full fat plain Greek yogurt
- ½ cup frozen strawberries
- 2 to 3 teaspoons monkfruit sweetener
- ½ teaspoon vanilla extract
- Pinch of salt
- Optional: 1 teaspoon lemon juice or 1 teaspoon allulose

Instructions

Blend until fully smooth. Taste and adjust sweetness. Freeze 2 to 3 hours until scoopable. Rest briefly before serving.

Mint Chip Nice Cream

Ingredients

- ½ cup full fat cottage cheese
- ½ cup full fat plain Greek yogurt
- 2 to 3 teaspoons monkfruit sweetener
- ¼ to ½ teaspoon peppermint extract
- 1 teaspoon vanilla extract
- Pinch of salt
- 2 tablespoons finely chopped dark chocolate
- Optional: 1 teaspoon allulose

Instructions

Blend everything except the chocolate until smooth. Freeze 1½ to 2 hours until thick. Fold in chocolate. Freeze an additional 30 to 60 minutes. Let soften slightly before scooping.

Chocolate Nice Cream

Ingredients

- ½ cup full fat cottage cheese
- ½ cup full fat plain Greek yogurt
- 2 to 3 teaspoons monkfruit sweetener
- 2 tablespoons unsweetened cocoa powder
- 1 teaspoon vanilla extract
- Pinch of salt
- Optional: 1 tablespoon melted dark chocolate or 1 teaspoon allulose

Instructions

Blend until silky smooth with no cocoa pockets. Taste and adjust sweetness. Freeze 2 to 3 hours until scoopable. Let rest briefly before serving.

Quick Sweet Treats

<u>Chocolate Chia Pudding</u>
Chia seeds mixed with almond milk, cocoa, monk fruit, and vanilla. Chill until thickened.

<u>Vanilla Chia Pudding</u>
Chia seeds mixed with almond milk, vanilla, and monk fruit. Chill overnight, then add berries.

<u>Berry Yogurt Parfait</u>
Greek yogurt layered with monk fruit, berries, and nuts.

<u>Protein Cookie Dough Bites</u>
Protein powder, almond flour, almond butter, monk fruit, and vanilla rolled into chilled bites.

<u>Yogurt with Almond Butter and Chocolate Shell</u>
Greek yogurt topped with almond butter and melted sugar-free chocolate mixed with a little coconut oil.

You don't have to go home, but....

Yvonne

Ending a big conversation at the table with a healthy meal is exactly how we wanted it. There is so much to take in, and our hope is that you reach for this book when you need it. Our even greater hope is that if you are healthy now, you never need this book as a resource for recovery.

Taura

Instead, may it spark a shift. We do not want to lead these statistics anymore. Stress, poor diets, lack of exercise, skipping checkups, and tuning out our own bodies have cost us too much already. The question on my fridge has become the question in my heart. Will this nourish me or harm me? If it is the latter, put it down, walk away, swear it off, or do whatever it takes. There is only one of you, and your next breath, your next laugh, your next hug, your next declaration to begin again is the gift of again. May you and your loved ones open it with intention, cherish it fully, and revel in its beauty.

Ashé

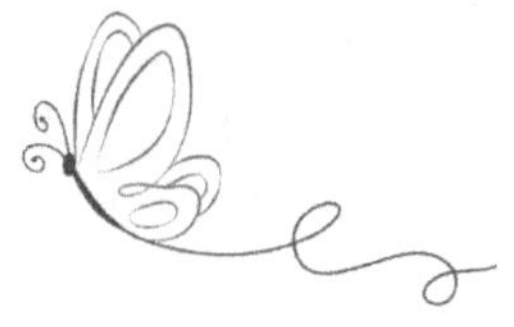

ACKNOWLEDGEMENTS

First of all, I want to thank my Lord and Savior, JESUS Christ, for saving me and for bringing me through this test. Thank GOD for blessing me with my beautiful, awesome, and gifted daughter, Taura. Without her love, care, and fantastic meals, I wouldn't have made it through my stroke recovery as well as I did. I love and appreciate her so much. Without Taura, this project, *THE GIFT OF AGAIN*, wouldn't exist.

I truly thank, love, admire, and appreciate our very own talented maestro extraordinaire, engineer and producer of our audiobook, Darien Dorsey. I also want to thank everyone who took time out of their busy lives to share their journeys with us. I thank GOD for their continued health and recovery.

Together, we want to thank our family in Birmingham, Alabama. My siblings and Taura's aunts and uncles, Patricia, Sandra & Rob, Leila Faye, Michael & Cheryl, Danny & Trishann, Sharmell, and all of their children and extended family. We would also like to acknowledge the siblings who have passed on: Vanessa, Kandi, and Jit.

Big love to our friends and framily in Oakland: Dennis Rhodes, the Stinsons, the Lothlens, the Pearsons, the Sumners, the Chavarins', and special thanks to Barbara McElhaney and the entire McElhaney family.

We want to collectively thank Mindy, Clarence McElhaney, Tymiak Hawkins, Tracey Brown, and Emiko Carlin. We are so grateful to you all for sharing your stroke survival stories. Thank you for the time and emotional investment you made into *THE GIFT OF AGAIN*. We also want to thank the medical professionals who contributed to this book: Jessica Brewer, Dr. Swati Laroia Coon, Dr. Kimberly Johnson Hatchett, and Jerome Lawrence. Thank you for sharing your expert advice with our readers with such commitment and care. Your words validate what we see in our communities every day. We're confident we can move the needle in the right direction together. Thank you again.

First and foremost, I want thank Jesus Christ for all that He's done and all that He's yet to do. I enjoy our talks, and I'm so thankful to hear you more clearly these days.

Tremendous gratitude, love, honor, respect and admiration to my Queen, my beautiful mother, Yvonne Stinson,

Thank you for sharing your story. It will help so many people, and quite honestly, your bravery and understanding have helped me in ways I cannot fully express. I am so blessed to open the gift of hearing your voice every day, and I do not take that for granted. May God give you the desires of your heart, Mom. You deserve it. I love you so much.

Also sending so much love, honor, and gratitude to my Dad, Willie Stinson! Thank you for your endless prayers, support, love, and transparency!

To my sister, Tanecia, thank you for your love, support, and friendship! Watching you grow from a baby to a woman with a baby of your own has been the best view I have ever seen. I'm so proud of you and I love you so much! And thanks to my nephew Xzavier, for being the brightest shining light. I can't wait to support you in whatever you do. I have a feeling it will be creative, my little singer-pianist.

To my brother Glen, who will always be ageless, we need your book next…And to Theresa, thank you for your love and support.

I love you all so much!

To my partner Darien, thank you for the morning coffee after nights of writing, and for being such a generous, kind, and supportive presence in my life. I love you beyond the moon, stars and mars…and only you know how much I love the cosmos. Thanks for always looking up with me! Many thanks as well to your beautiful parents, Mr. & Mrs Dorsey! Beautiful parts of each of you is the perfect recipe that makes up Darien Dorsey! So funny, focused, smart, kind, and talented! Thank you both for your prayers, kindness and prayers. Big love to OUR brother Kevin..your podcast and cookbook is already in demand. Give the people what they want! IJS☺

Sending big love to our tribe, starting with the smallest and most talented, my niece Zirah, one of my favorite people on earth, alongside her parents and my ANCHORS, my brostie Charles Kelley, and my Sistie Quiana…love you four, deep. We can't forget my furry niece, Luga Mae.

To my beautiful best friend since fifth grade, Kyra Dyas, and her mom, Viola Louise Dyas, who tried to tell us so much of what is in this book back when we just wanted sugary cereal. I love you!

Big love to my beautiful sister Brély Evans, who has walked this path with me since high school. God knew then, and He's not finished with us yet…I love you! So thankful to have started this journey with you and Mykah Montgomery…love you Mykie.

Also, big love to everyone in B210, especially Roxanne Ross Barlow and Gillian Ovid, whose love and laughter carry me more than they know. Odessa, Allecia, Nyjeri, Delanie and Lailah, I will never forget the beautiful times, lessons learned and the love and laughter we shared during our becoming years. Also thanks to Kesha Joyner for your endless support, and to Delanie West…forever east coast 210. I love you all.

Adama Wilson, I miss you more than any word could express. Even six years later, I am routinely, a total mess, but then I feel your love, or hear your voice telling me to pick myself up in only a way that you can, and I am better, for the moment. Huge love to the Wilson Family. Auntie Rhita, Uncle Claude, My homie…Ayanna and Maya.

I love you all so much!

Biggest love to Candace Coles Georges, my sister, the joy maker. I love you and Chris so much! Major and Nichelle Johnson (BOND), our game nights give me life more than you all know!

Ray Ray, I love you.

Laura and Nora, "we're in this life together," is one of the moments I will always go back to for an emotional refresh. I love you both.

Also, lots of love to my sister and dear friend Carolyn Richardson, who can drown darkness with her light with one hand and give you delicious chocolates with the other…love you!

Nick, my Bro-tell. Thank you for always being so protective of me and being a true friend.

Lots of love to Jamie Hawkins for a lifetime of friendship and prayers.

Big love to my friends and collaborators, Allyson Newman and Heather McIntosh(So-so good), Khiyon Hursey, Jack Dolgen, as well as as my partners in change at AMPAS, THE BLACK CAUCUS, THE AWFC, and my incredible team, Stephanie Slangs, and Jeff Jernigan, andlooking forward to so many things with both of you, we have lots of road ahead of us! Also many thanks to Carli Haney…looking forward to building with you and thanks so much for giving me a home BACE to ride at…and thanks the eternal sunshine that is Cara Chambrello!

Also, to my family mentioned above, there are a few I want to personally acknowledge: my two-fer, my suzzin and cuzstie, Nadia Tellis, and my suzzins Phadyra Collier Foster and Charlena Morton. My Bruzzin - Darryl Morton, Rell, Preacher and all of my first cousins on both sides, I love you all.

My sister-cousin Brittni Lothlen Jackson, thank you for your endless support and FaceTimes. I love you and all of your siblings like they were my own. Leonard Lothlen Jr. Mariah, you are so naturally talented…show the world ho naturally funny you are…so glad we byke…love you so much. Dr. Joya Chavarin…I am so proud of you!

Also lots of love and cherished memories to my cousins Patria Dye, Kalila Rafa, Wendy, Aaron and Nyka Grayson. Cerlia…thank you for all that you do for Grandma and just for being a bright and positive light!

If I added every name from both sides, I would go over the character allotment, so in closing, I want to thank my Grandma Grace, who, at 97 years young, is so witty, funny, and emotionally and spiritually present. I can't wait for the 100th birthday celebration.

Love you, Grandma. And she'd say, "Love you more."

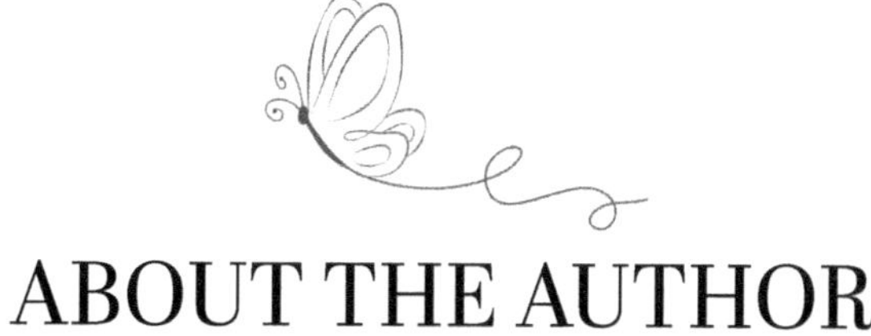

ABOUT THE AUTHOR

Yvonne Stinson is a creative and entrepreneur whose life has always been rooted in care, artistry, and community. A celebrated hairstylist in Oakland, California, she also founded Joyful Celebrations, a singing telegram and children's party company built on bringing joy to others. She also served as a special needs educator, extending her gift of care into the classroom. Yvonne has a gift for creating something out of nothing, whether with a needle and thread, butter and flour, or her voice. A poet currently working on her first collection, she remains deeply connected to her community, spending her time caring for others, baking, and being with family.

Taura Stinson is a natural born storyteller who began writing at eight years old, when her mother placed a composition notebook in her hands to harness her wild imagination. When her late uncle, a songwriter, read her early work, he gave a name to the constant stream of ideas pouring out of her. Songs. She went on to become a Critics Choice and SCL Award winning, Oscar, Golden Globe, Emmy, and Grammy nominated songwriter, and the author of the five star, beloved book, *100 THINGS EVERY BLACK GIRL SHOULD KNOW*. Born in Alabama and raised in Oakland, she now resides in Los Angeles, where she advocates for underserved voices and continues to create music and narrative driven stories for television and film.

SOURCES

Preface

100 Black Men of America. Health & Wellness. https://100black-men.org/four-for-the-future/health-wellness

Association of Black Cardiologists. Cardiovascular disease prevention and treatment resources. https://www.abcardio.org

Black Women's Health Imperative. Health advocacy for Black women and girls. https://bwhi.org

Centers for Disease Control and Prevention. Stroke Facts. https://www.cdc.gov/stroke/data-research/facts-stats/index.html

Curtin SC. Trends in Stroke Death Rates: United States, 2000–2022. NCHS Data Brief No. 505. National Center for Health Statistics. August 2024. https://www.cdc.gov/nchs/products/databriefs/db505.htm

Martin SS, Aday AW, Almarzooq ZI, et al. 2024 Heart Disease and Stroke Statistics. Circulation. 2024;149:e347–e913. doi:10.1161/CIR.0000000000001209

National Alliance for Hispanic Health. Science-based health resources for Hispanic communities. https://www.healthyamericas.org

National Black Nurses Association. Health advocacy for Black and underserved communities. https://nbna.org

National Hispanic Medical Association. Improving health outcomes for Hispanic and underserved communities. https://www.nhmamd. org

U.S. Department of Health and Human Services, Office of Minority Health. Heart disease and Asian Americans. https://minorityhealth. hhs.gov/heart-disease-and-asian-americans

U.S. Department of Health and Human Services, Office of Minority Health. Stroke and Black/African Americans. https://minorityhealth. hhs.gov/stroke-and-blackafrican-americans

WomenHeart: The National Coalition for Women with Heart Disease. https://www.womenheart.org

Chapter One

American Heart Association. Cold Weather and Cardiovascular Disease. https://www.heart.org/en/health-topics/consumer-healthcare/what-is-cardiovascular-disease/cold-weather-and-cardiovascular-disease

American Stroke Association. Let's Talk About Black Americans and Stroke. https://www.stroke.org/en/help-and-support/resource-library/lets-talk-about-stroke/black-americans

American Stroke Association. Let's Talk About Hispanic and Latino Americans and Stroke. https://www.stroke.org/en/help-and-support/resource-library/lets-talk-about-stroke/hispanic-and-latino-americans

American Stroke Association. Let's Talk About Transient Ischemic Attack (TIA). https://www.stroke.org/en/help-and-support/resource-library/lets-talk-about-stroke/transient-ischemic-attack

American Stroke Association. Let's Talk About Stroke — Types of Stroke. https://www.stroke.org/en/about-stroke/types-of-stroke

Association of Asian Pacific Community Health Organizations (AAP-CHO). Health advocacy for Asian Americans, Native Hawaiians, and Pacific Islanders. https://aapcho.org

Bhaskaran K, et al. Short term effects of temperature on risk of myocardial infarction in England and Wales. BMJ. 2010;341:c3823. doi:10.1136/bmj.c3823

Go Red for Women. American Heart Association. Heart disease and stroke resources for women. https://www.goredforwomen.org

Chapter Four

American Stroke Association. Diabetes and Stroke Prevention. https://www.stroke.org/en/about-stroke/stroke-risk-factors/diabetes-and-stroke-prevention

Brill JB. Cholesterol Down. New York: Three Rivers Press; 2006.

Buettner D. The Blue Zones. Washington, DC: National Geographic Society; 2008.

DerrameCerebral.org. Spanish-language stroke prevention and awareness. American Stroke Association. https://www.derramecerebral.org

Foundation for Black Women's Wellness. Heart health education for Black women and families. https://www.ffbww.org

Harvard Health Publishing. Can you lengthen your life? Harvard Health Letter. https://www.health.harvard.edu

Hispanic Community Health Study / Study of Latinos (HCHS/SOL). National Heart, Lung, and Blood Institute. https://www.nhlbi.nih.gov/science/hispanic-community-health-studystudy-latinos-hchssol

Hjelmborg JV, et al. Genetic influence on human lifespan and longevity. Human Genetics. 2006;119(3):312–321. doi:10.1007/s00439-006-0144-y

Lincoff AM, et al. Semaglutide and cardiovascular outcomes in obesity without diabetes. New England Journal of Medicine. 2023;389(24):2221–2232. doi:10.1056/NEJMoa2307563

National Heart, Lung, and Blood Institute. Your Heart, Your Life — heart health resources for the Hispanic/Latino community. https://www.nhlbi.nih.gov/education/heart-truth/CHW/YHYL

Chapter Five

Amarenco P, et al. One-year risk of stroke after transient ischemic attack or minor stroke. New England Journal of Medicine. 2016;374(16):1533–1542. doi:10.1056/NEJMoa1412981

American Diabetes Association. Stroke Prevention. https://diabetes.org/about-diabetes/complications/stroke

American Heart Association. Heart Disease and Stroke Statistics Fact Sheet: Asian Race and Cardiovascular Diseases. Available in Chinese, Hindi, Ilocano, and other languages. https://www.heart.org/en/about-us/heart-and-stroke-association-statistics

American Stroke Association. Let's Talk About the Connection Between Diabetes and Stroke. https://www.stroke.org/en/help-and-support/resource-library/lets-talk-about-stroke/diabetes

Buettner D. The Blue Zones. Washington, DC: National Geographic Society; 2008.

Buettner D, Skemp S. Blue Zones: Lessons from the World's Longest Lived. American Journal of Lifestyle Medicine. 2016;10(5):318–321. doi:10.1177/1559827616637066

Buettner D. Blue Zones Kitchen: 100 Recipes to Live to 100. Washington, DC: National Geographic; 2019.

Emerging Risk Factors Collaboration. Diabetes mellitus, fasting blood glucose, and risk of vascular disease. Lancet. 2010;375(9733):2215–2222. doi:10.1016/S0140-6736(10)60484-9

Erlangsen A, Runeson B, Bolton JM, et al. Association between spousal suicide and mental, physical, and social health outcomes. JAMA Psychiatry. 2017;74(5):456–464. doi:10.1001/jamapsychiatry.2017.0226

HispanicHealth.info. Health resources in English and Spanish. National Hispanic Medical Association. https://hispanichealth.info

Li J, Johansen C, Hansen D, Olsen J. Cancer incidence in parents who lost a child: a nationwide study in Denmark. Cancer. 2002;95(10):2237–2242. doi:10.1002/cncr.10943

Li J, Precht DH, Mortensen PB, Olsen J. Mortality in parents after death of a child in Denmark. Lancet. 2003;361(9355):363–367. doi:10.1016/S0140-6736(03)12387-2

Longo VD, Mattson MP. Fasting: molecular mechanisms and clinical applications. Cell Metabolism. 2014;19(2):181–192. doi:10.1016/j.cmet.2013.12.008

Longo VD, Anderson RM. Caloric restriction, intermittent fasting, and longevity. Cell. 2022;185(11):1914–1932. doi:10.1016/j.cell.2022.04.002

Longo V. The Longevity Diet. New York: Avery; 2018.

National Hispanic Health Foundation. Leadership, research, and education to improve Hispanic health equity. https://nationalhispanichealthfoundation.org

Women's Heart Alliance. Advocacy and resources for heart disease as the leading killer of women. https://womensheartalliance.org

Chapter Seven

American Heart Association. Stress and heart health. https://www.heart.org/en/healthy-living/healthy-lifestyle/stress-management/stress-and-heart-health

Appel LJ, et al. A clinical trial of the effects of dietary patterns on blood pressure. New England Journal of Medicine. 1997;336(16):1117–1124. doi:10.1056/NEJM199704173361601

Association of Asian Pacific Community Health Organizations (AAP-CHO). Advocacy and health resources for Asian Americans, Native Hawaiians, and Pacific Islanders. https://aapcho.org

Bushnell C, Howard VJ, Lisabeth L, et al. Sex differences in the evaluation and treatment of acute ischaemic stroke. Lancet Neurology. 2018;17(7):641–650. doi:10.1016/S1474-4422(18)30201-1

Davis DR, Epp MD, Riordan HD. Changes in USDA food composition data for 43 garden crops, 1950 to 1999. Journal of the American College of Nutrition. 2004;23(6):669–682. doi:10.1080/07315724.2004.10719409

Dawson J, et al. Vagus nerve stimulation paired with rehabilitation for upper limb motor function after ischaemic stroke (VNS-RE-HAB). Lancet. 2021;397(10284):1545–1553. doi:10.1016/S0140-6736(21)00475-X

Deichmann R, Lavie C, Andrews S. Coenzyme Q10 and statin-induced mitochondrial dysfunction. Ochsner Journal. 2010;10(1):16–21.

Feigin VL, et al. Global, regional, and national burden of stroke and its risk factors, 1990–2019. Lancet Neurology. 2021;20(10):795–820. doi:10.1016/S1474-4422(21)00252-0

Go Red for Women. Stroke and heart disease awareness for women. American Heart Association. https://www.goredforwomen.org

Jackson CA, Sudlow CLM, Mishra GD. Psychological distress and risk of myocardial infarction and stroke. Circulation: Cardiovascular Quality and Outcomes. 2018;11(9):e004500. doi:10.1161/CIRCOUTCOMES.117.004500

Littarru GP, Tiano L. Bioenergetic and antioxidant properties of coenzyme Q10: recent developments. Molecular Biotechnology. 2007;37(1):31–37. doi:10.1007/s12033-007-0052-y

Martínez Steele E, et al. Ultra-processed foods and added sugars in the US diet. BMJ Open. 2016;6(3):e009892. doi:10.1136/bmjopen-2015-009892

National Heart, Lung, and Blood Institute. DASH Eating Plan. https://www.nhlbi.nih.gov/education/dash-eating-plan

National Heart, Lung, and Blood Institute. MOSAAIC Study — cardiovascular health research in Asian American and Pacific Islander communities. https://www.nhlbi.nih.gov/news/2024/new-nhlbi-study-focuses-asian-americans-native-hawaiians-and-pacific-islanders

Reddin C, et al. Association of psychosocial stress with risk of acute stroke. JAMA Network Open. 2022;5(12):e2244836. doi:10.1001/jamanetworkopen.2022.44836

Rosman L, et al. Posttraumatic stress disorder and risk for stroke in young and middle-aged adults. Stroke. 2019;50(11):2996–3003. doi:10.1161/STROKEAHA.119.025808

Rusek M, et al. Ketogenic diet in Alzheimer's disease. International Journal of Molecular Sciences. 2019;20(16):3892. doi:10.3390/ijms20163892

U.S. Department of Health and Human Services, Office of Minority Health. Heart disease and Hispanic Americans. https://minorityhealth.hhs.gov/heart-disease-and-hispanic-americans

Włodarek D. Role of ketogenic diets in neurodegenerative diseases. Nutrients. 2019;11(1):169. doi:10.3390/nu11010169

WomenHeart: The National Coalition for Women with Heart Disease. https://www.womenheart.org

World Stroke Organization. Global Stroke Fact Sheet 2025. https://www.world-stroke.org/world-stroke-day-campaign/why-stroke-matters/learn-about-stroke

Chapter Eight

American Stroke Association. Smoking and Stroke. https://www.stroke.org/en/about-stroke/stroke-risk-factors/stroke-risk-factors-under-your-control/smoking-and-stroke

American Stroke Association. Women and Stroke — unique risk factors and prevention. https://www.stroke.org/en/about-stroke/stroke-risk-factors/stroke-risk-factors-not-within-your-control/women-and-stroke

Estruch R, et al. Primary prevention of cardiovascular disease with a Mediterranean diet (PREDIMED Trial). New England Journal of Medicine. 2018;378(25):e34. doi:10.1056/NEJMoa1800389

Ettehad D, et al. Blood pressure lowering for prevention of cardiovascular disease and death. Lancet. 2016;387(10022):957–967. doi:10.1016/S0140-6736(15)01225-8

GBD 2021 Stroke Risk Factor Collaborators. Global, regional, and national burden of stroke and its risk factors, 1990–2021. Lancet Neurology. 2024. doi:10.1016/S1474-4422(24)00369-7

Hackshaw A, et al. Low cigarette consumption and risk of coronary heart disease and stroke. BMJ. 2018;360:j5855. doi:10.1136/bmj.j5855

Hispanic Community Health Study / Study of Latinos (HCHS/SOL). National Heart, Lung, and Blood Institute. https://www.nhlbi.nih.gov/science/hispanic-community-health-studystudy-latinos-hchssol

Hutton C, et al. Polygenic risk, midlife Life's Simple 7, and lifetime risk of stroke. Journal of the American Heart Association. 2022;11(15):e025703. doi:10.1161/JAHA.122.025703

Katan M, Luft A. Global burden of stroke. Seminars in Neurology. 2018;38(2):208–211. doi:10.1055/s-0038-1649503

Ling C, Rönn T. Epigenetics in human obesity and type 2 diabetes. Cell Metabolism. 2019;29(5):1028–1044. doi:10.1016/j.cmet.2019.03.009

Martínez-González MA, Gea A, Ruiz-Canela M. The Mediterranean diet and cardiovascular health. Circulation Research. 2019;124(5):779–798. doi:10.1161/CIRCRESAHA.118.313348

National Black Nurses Association. Health advocacy and resources for Black and underserved communities. https://nbna.org

O'Donnell MJ, et al. Global and regional effects of potentially modifiable risk factors associated with acute stroke in 32 countries (INTERSTROKE). Lancet. 2016;388(10046):761–775. doi:10.1016/S0140-6736(16)30506-2

Ornish D, et al. Changes in prostate gene expression in men undergoing an intensive nutrition and lifestyle intervention. Proceedings of the National Academy of Sciences. 2008;105(24):8369–8374. doi:10.1073/pnas.0803080105

PROGRESS Collaborative Group. Randomised trial of a perindopril-based blood-pressure-lowering regimen. Lancet. 2001;358(9287):1033–1041. doi:10.1016/S0140-6736(01)06178-5

Rutten-Jacobs LC, et al. Genetic risk, incident stroke, and the benefits of adhering to a healthy lifestyle: cohort study of 306,473 UK Biobank participants. BMJ. 2018;363:k4168. doi:10.1136/bmj.k4168

U.S. Department of Health and Human Services, Office of Minority Health. Heart disease and Asian Americans. https://minorityhealth.hhs.gov/heart-disease-and-asian-americans

Women's Heart Alliance. Advocacy and resources dedicated to women's heart health. https://womensheartalliance.org

Chapter Nine

American Diabetes Association. Glycemic Index and Diabetes. https://diabetes.org/food-nutrition/understanding-carbs/glycemic-index-and-diabetes

American Heart Association. Saturated Fats. https://www.heart.org/en/healthy-living/healthy-eating/eat-smart/fats/saturated-fats

American Heart Association. Sodium and Salt. https://www.heart.org/en/healthy-living/healthy-eating/eat-smart/sodium/sodium-and-salt

American Heart Association. Trans Fats. https://www.heart.org/en/healthy-living/healthy-eating/eat-smart/fats/trans-fat

Association of Asian Pacific Community Health Organizations (AAPCHO). Nutrition and health resources for Asian Americans, Native Hawaiians, and Pacific Islanders. https://aapcho.org

DerrameCerebral.org. Spanish-language stroke prevention and nutrition resources. https://www.derramecerebral.org

Foundation for Black Women's Wellness. Heart health and nutrition programs for Black women. https://www.ffbww.org

HispanicHealth.info. Nutrition and health resources in English and Spanish. https://hispanichealth.info

National Institutes of Health, MedlinePlus. Dietary Fats. https://medlineplus.gov/dietaryfats.html

U.S. Food and Drug Administration. Added Sugars on the New Nutrition Facts Label. https://www.fda.gov/food/new-nutrition-facts-label/added-sugars-new-nutrition-facts-label

U.S. Food and Drug Administration. How to Understand and Use the Nutrition Facts Label. https://www.fda.gov/food/new-nutrition-facts-label/how-understand-and-use-nutrition-facts-label

U.S. Food and Drug Administration. Trans Fat. https://www.fda.gov/food/food-additives-petitions/trans-fat

USDA FoodData Central. National Nutrient Database. U.S. Department of Agriculture. https://fdc.nal.usda.gov

WomenHeart: The National Coalition for Women with Heart Disease. https://www.womenheart.org